Neurochemical Basis of Brain Function and Dysfunction

Edited by Thomas Heinbockel and Antonei B. Csoka

Published in London, United Kingdom

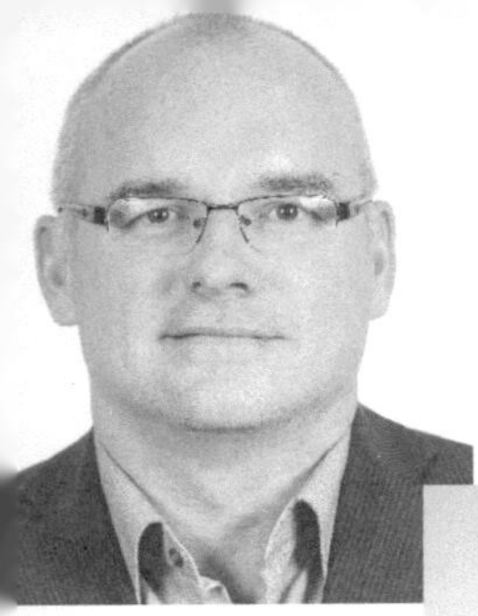
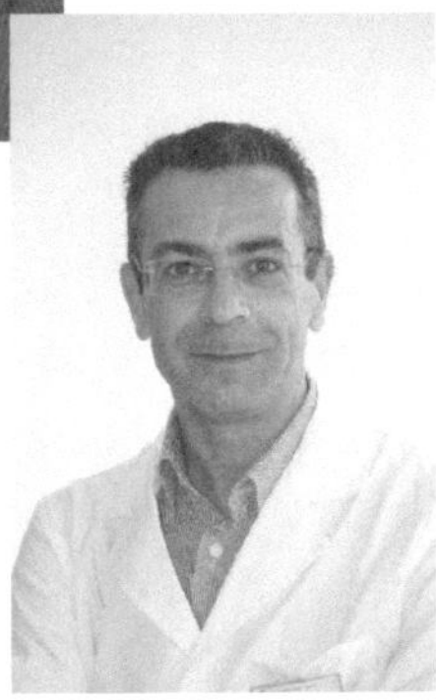
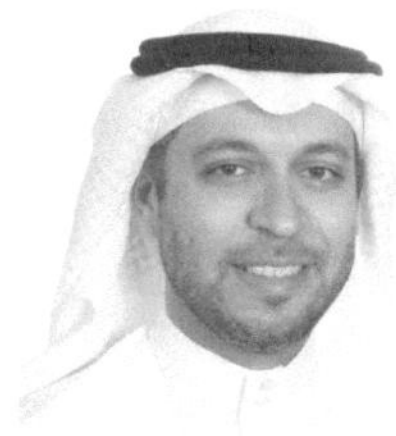
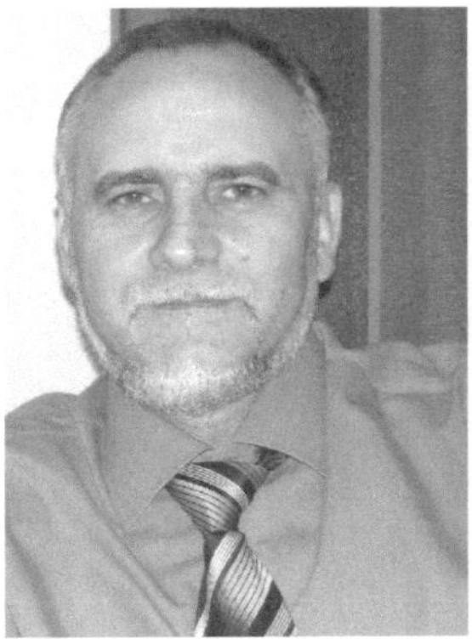
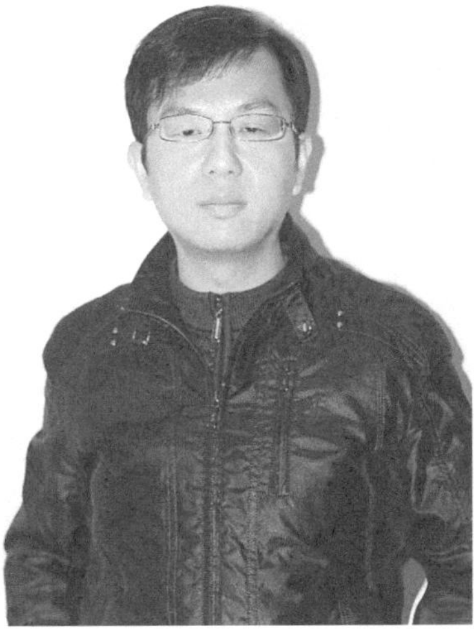
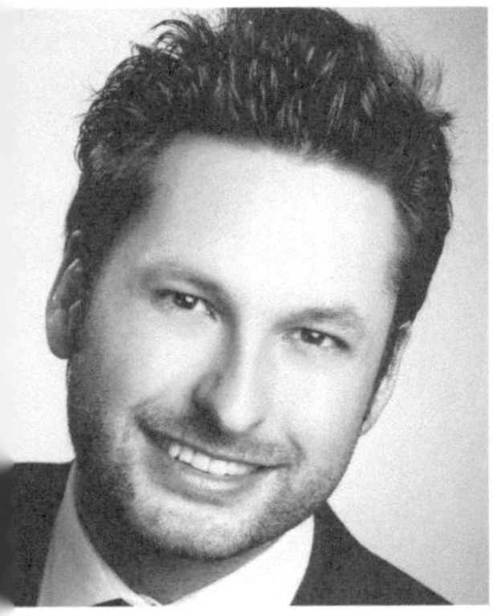
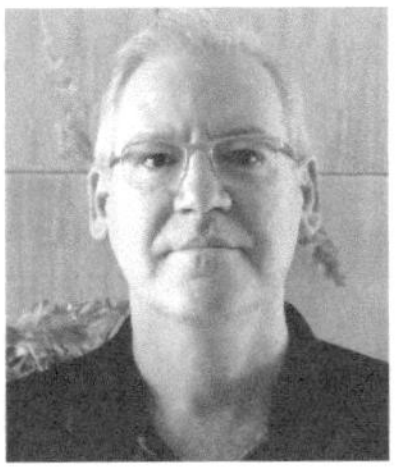

IntechOpen

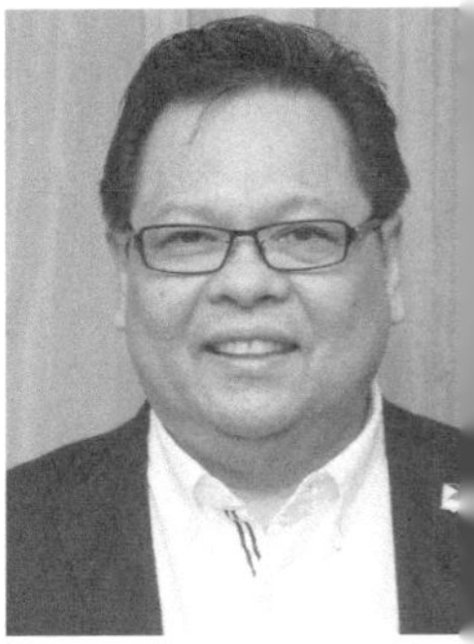
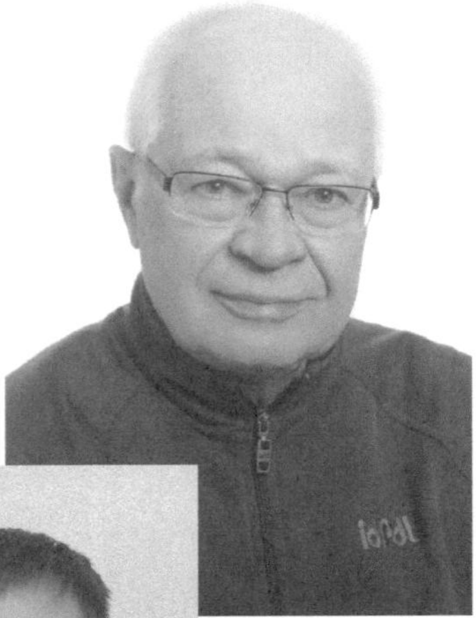
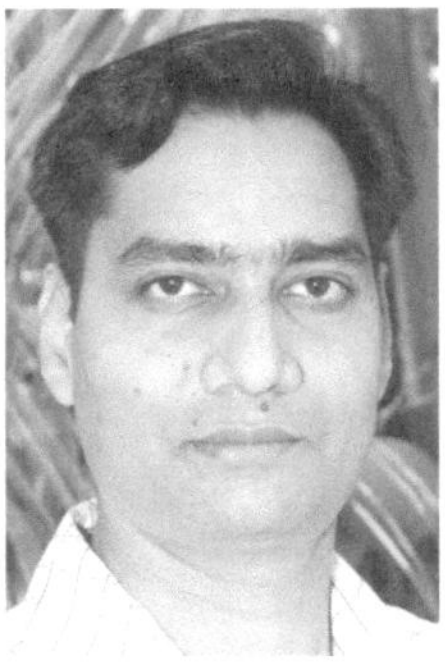
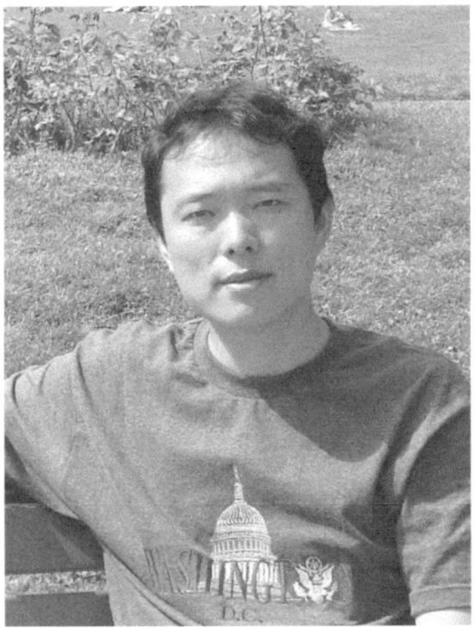
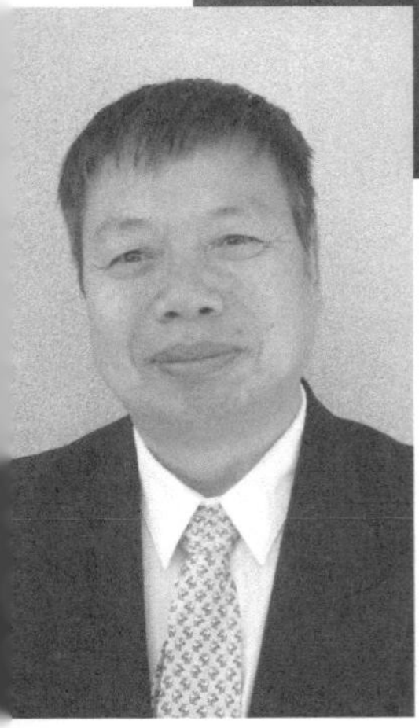
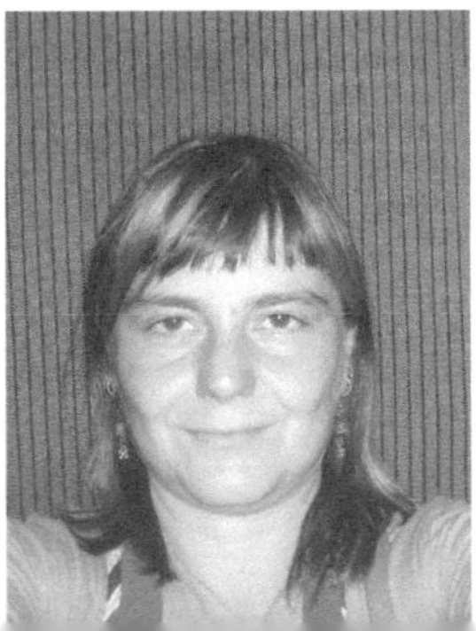

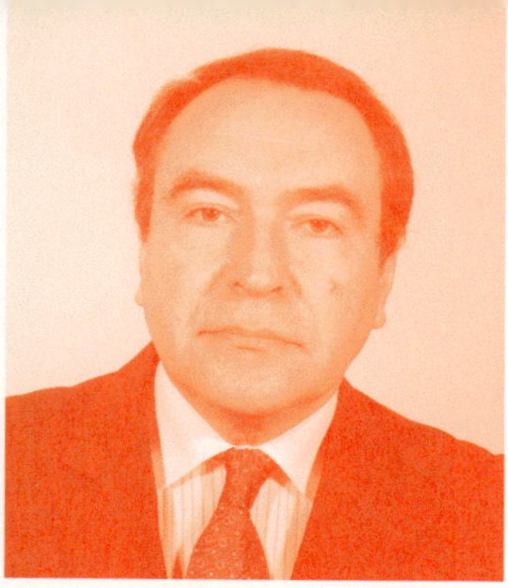
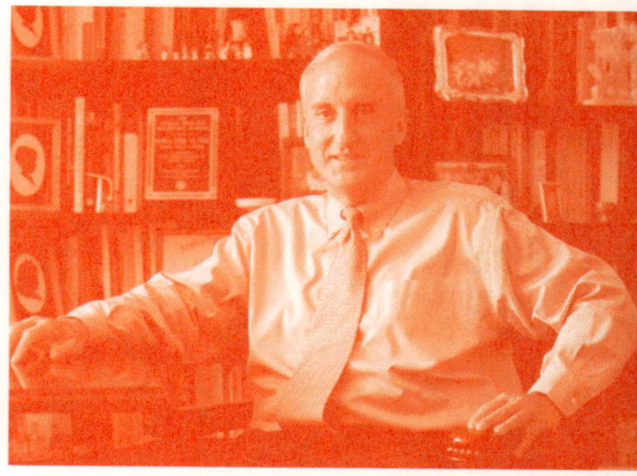
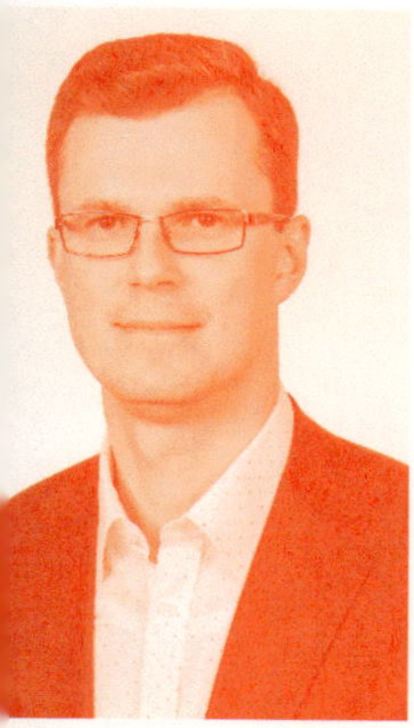
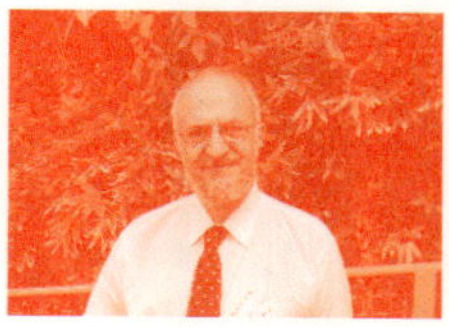
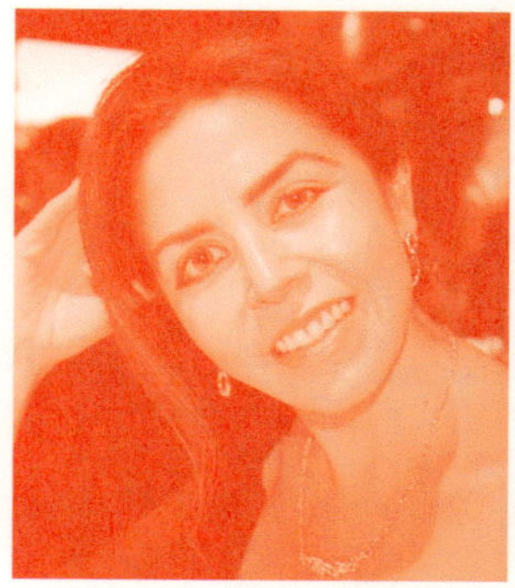

Supporting open minds since 2005

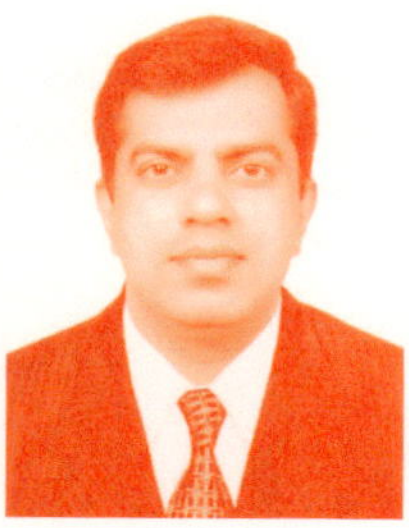
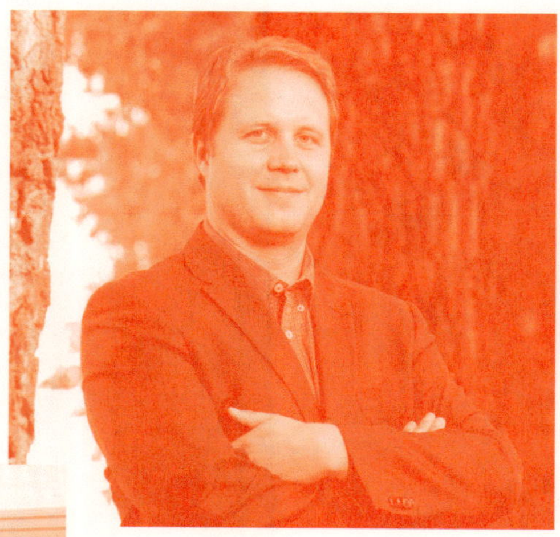
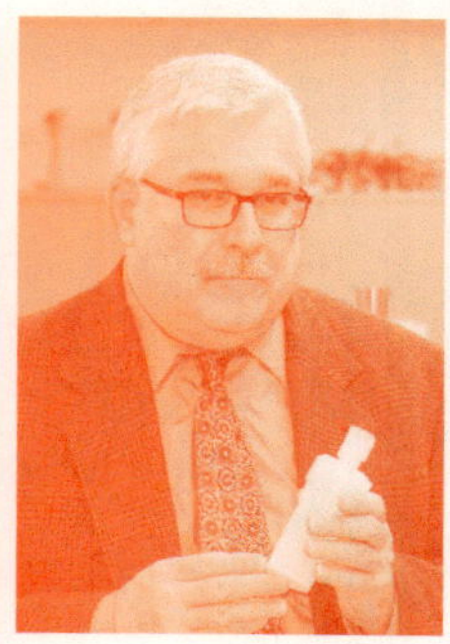
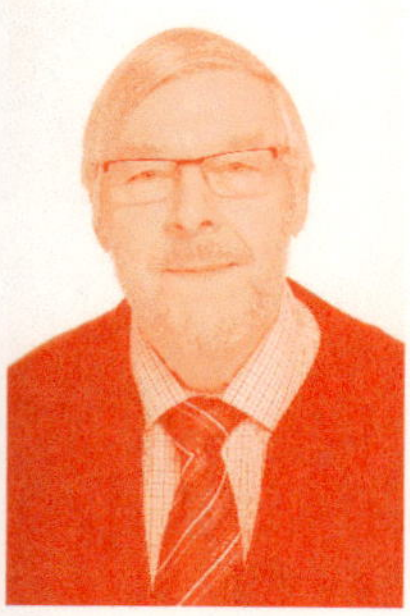
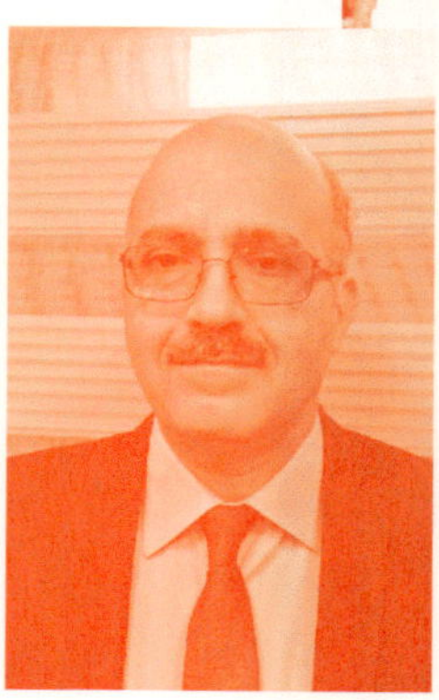
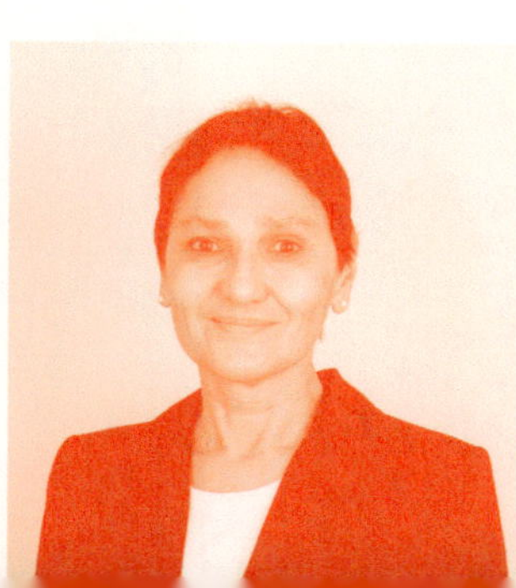
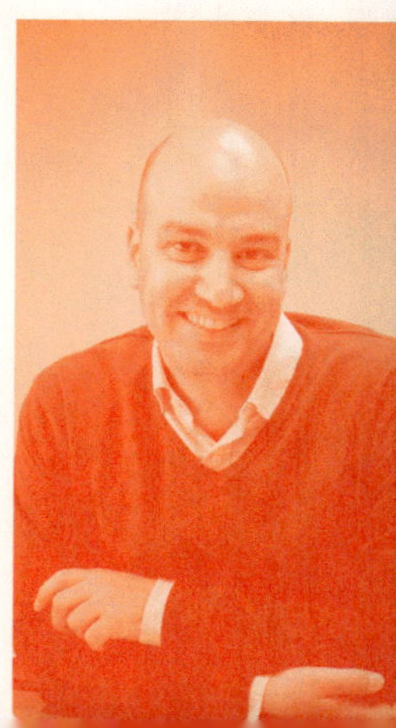

Neurochemical Basis of Brain Function and Dysfunction
http://dx.doi.org/10.5772/intechopen.75850
Edited by Thomas Heinbockel and Antonei B. Csoka

Contributors
Abdulbaki Agbas, Shi-Xian Deng, Jole Fiorito, Ottavio Arancio, Donald W. Landry, Manorama Patri, Thomas Heinbockel, Antonei B. Csoka

First published in London, United Kingdom, 2019 by IntechOpen
IntechOpen is the global imprint of INTECHOPEN LIMITED, registered in England and Wales, registration number: 11086078, The Shard, 25th floor, 32 London Bridge Street
London, SE19SG – United Kingdom
Printed in Croatia

British Library Cataloguing-in-Publication Data
A catalogue record for this book is available from the British Library

Additional hard and PDF copies can be obtained from orders@intechopen.com

Neurochemical Basis of Brain Function and Dysfunction
Edited by Thomas Heinbockel and Antonei B. Csoka
p. cm.
Print ISBN 978-1-78985-999-7
Online ISBN 978-1-83880-000-0
eBook (PDF) ISBN 978-1-83880-025-3

Meet the editors

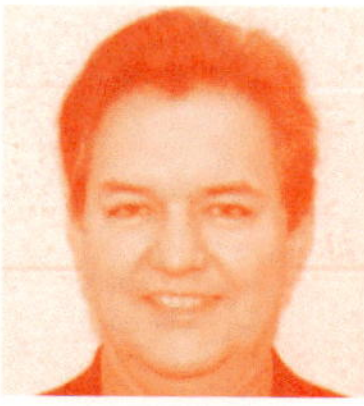

Thomas Heinbockel, PhD, is Professor and Interim Chair in the Department of Anatomy, Howard University College of Medicine, Washington, DC. Dr. Heinbockel's laboratory engages in multidisciplinary research to elucidate organizational principles of neural systems in the brain, specifically the limbic and olfactory system. His research has been directed at understanding brain mechanisms of information processing and their relation to neurological and neuropsychiatric disorders. His lab works also on translational projects, specifically the development of novel anti-epileptic drugs and pharmacotherapeutic treatment options for drug addiction. His lab analyzes drug actions at the epi and genetic levels using next-generation sequencing technology. Dr. Heinbockel studied biology at the Philipps-University, Marburg, Germany. His studies of the brain started during his MS thesis work at the Max-Planck-Institute for Behavioral Physiology, Starnberg/Seewiesen, Germany. Subsequently, he completed a PhD in Neuroscience at the University of Arizona, Tucson, Arizona, USA. After graduating, he was a Research Associate at the Institute of Physiology, Otto-von-Guericke-University School of Medicine, Magdeburg, Germany. Prior to his arrival at Howard University, Dr. Heinbockel held joint research faculty appointments in the Department of Anatomy and Neurobiology and the Department of Physiology at the University of Maryland School of Medicine, Baltimore, Maryland, USA. He still maintains an adjunct appointment in these departments.

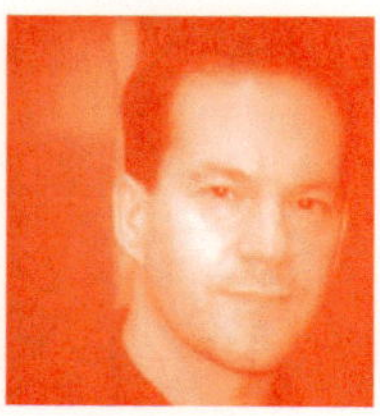

Antonei B. Csoka, PhD is Associate Professor in the Department of Anatomy at Howard University, Washington, DC, where he directs the Epigenetics Laboratory. Dr. Csoka received his BS in Genetics from the University of Newcastle, UK, his MS in Molecular Pathology from the University of Leicester, UK, and his PhD in Cell and Molecular Biology from the University of Debrecen, Hungary. He performed postdoctoral research at the University of California, San Francisco, where he cloned the human hyaluronidase genes. At Brown University, he was a member of the team that identified the causative gene for Hutchinson-Gilford Progeria Syndrome (Progeria), a disease with many features of "accelerated aging." At Howard, Dr. Csoka is studying the role of cellular senescence in human aging and the role of epigenetics in pharmacology and neuroscience.

Contents

Preface

Neurochemistry is a vitally important academic discipline that contributes to our understanding of molecular, cellular, and medical neurobiology. As a field, neurochemistry focuses on the role of the chemical entities that build the nervous system, the function of neurons and glial cells in health and disease, aspects of cell metabolism and neurotransmission, and degenerative processes and aging of the nervous system. Accordingly, this book contains chapters on a variety of topics, written by experts in their respective fields. This book is a valuable resource for neurochemists and other scientists alike. In addition, it contributes to the training of current and future neurochemists and, hopefully, will lead us on the path to curing some of the biggest challenges in human health.

In Chapter 1 ('Introductory Chapter: The Chemical Basis of Neural Function and Dysfunction'), Drs. Thomas Heinbockel and Antonei Csoka introduce the field of neurochemistry as a whole. Holistically it is concerned with the types, structures, and functions of the chemical components of the nervous system, and how the physiology of the nervous system is regulated by said chemicals. Neurological diseases such as Alzheimer's and Parkinson's disease are often a consequence of changes in the body's neurochemistry. Medicine uses neurochemicals to alter brain function and treat disease. Neurochemists study how the components of the nervous system function during processes such as neural plasticity, neural development, and learning and memory formation, and how these components undergo changes during disease, neural dysfunction, and aging. The chapter also includes examples of how external and internal factors impact and modify neurochemistry.

In Chapter 2 ('Synaptic Transmission and Amino Acid Neurotransmitters'), Dr. Manorama Patri reviews the role of amino acids acting as neurotransmitters in the brain. Amino acids, primarily glutamic acid, GABA, aspartic acid, and glycine are released from pre-synaptic nerve terminals in response to action potentials and cross the synaptic cleft to bind with specific receptors on the postsynaptic membrane to elicit responses. Interestingly, unlike the monoamine transmitters (5% of the total synapses in brain), glutamate and GABA are thought to account for at least 50% of the synapses. Also, glutamate and aspartate in particular provide the CNS with many functions essential for learning and memory, structural and functional organisation, neural development, and neurodegeneration.

In Chapter 3 ('Trends of Protein Aggregation in Neurodegenerative Diseases') Dr. Abdulbaki Agbas introduces the reader to protein aggregations that occur in the brain and, thereby, cause neurodegenerative diseases. He outlines the nature of protein aggregation and proteolytic systems such as the proteasome and autophagosome in Alzheimer's disease, Parkinson's disease, amyotrophic lateral sclerosis, frontotemporal lobar degeneration, Huntington disease, and prion disease, including new studies and findings.

Finally, in Chapter 4 ('Targeting the NO/cGMP/CREB Phosphorylation Signaling Pathway in Alzheimer's Disease'), Dr. Jole Fiorito and colleagues provide a comprehensive review of the nitric oxide (NO) signaling pathway in the hippocampus and its role in the pathogenesis of Alzheimer's disease. This pathway culminates with the phosphorylation of the transcriptional factor cAMP-responsive element binding (CREB) protein via increase of cyclic guanosine monosphosphate (cGMP) and activation of cGMP-dependent protein kinase. The chapter provides an overview of the progress being made in modulating hippocampal synaptic transmissions, which are critical for learning and memory, by targeting different components of said pathway. Furthermore, the chapter explores recent research on the pathway through the use of phosphodiesterase inhibitors.

We are grateful to IntechOpen for conceiving of this book project and for asking us to serve as editors. Thanks goes to Dolores Kuzelj at IntechOpen for guiding us through the publication process and for moving the book ahead in a timely fashion. Thanks are also due to all contributors of this book for taking the time to write a chapter proposal, compose the chapter, and make the requested revisions. Hopefully all contributors will continue their neurochemistry research with many intellectual challenges in exciting new directions. T.H. would like to thank his wife Dr. Vonnie D.C. Shields, Associate Dean and Professor, Towson University, Towson, MD, and their son Torben Heinbockel for the time that he was able to spend working on this book project during the past year. Finally, T.H. is grateful to his parents Erich and Renate Heinbockel for their continuous support and interest in his work over many years.

Thomas Heinbockel, Ph.D.
Professor & Interim Chair,
Department of Anatomy,
Howard University College of Medicine,
Washington, DC, USA

Antonei B. Csoka, Ph.D.
Associate Professor,
Department of Anatomy,
Howard University College of Medicine,
Washington, DC, USA

Chapter 1

Introductory Chapter: The Chemical Basis of Neural Function and Dysfunction

Thomas Heinbockel and Antonei B. Csoka

1. Introduction

What is neurochemistry? As a field of study, neurochemistry is concerned with the types, structures and functions of the chemical components found in the nervous system [1]. These components in turn regulate the physiology of the nervous system [2–4]. Neurochemistry is mainly concerned with the chemicals that are specifically found in the nervous system such as small organic molecules, neurotransmitters and neuropeptides. Neurological diseases are often a reflection of changes in the body's neurochemistry, e.g., in Alzheimer's disease or Parkinson's disease. Medicine uses neurochemicals to alter brain function and treat disease. Neurochemists study how the components of the nervous system are at work during processes such as neural plasticity, neural development, learning and memory formation and how these components undergo changes during disease processes, neural dysfunction, and aging. This chapter will introduce the chemical components of the nervous system and briefly discuss how external and internal factors impact and modify these components.

2. Building blocks of the nervous system

The nervous system comprises a vast array of cells that vary in form and function and how they interact with other cells. The two principal types of cells are nerve cells or neurons and glial cells. Both types have many subtypes that are named based either on their shape or function. Neurons can be broadly classified as unipolar, bipolar, multipolar or pseudounipolar based on their arrangement and presence of dendrites and axons, or they are classified as sensory, motor or interneurons based on their function in neural networks. Dendrites are considered as the recipient portion of a nerve cell while axons carry information to other parts of the nervous system. However, this distinction can be blurred in neural circuits where both axons and dendrites can serve in either function. Axons reach a length of 1.5 m in adult humans and are even longer in larger animals such as giraffes. While axons serve as long-distance communication devices for information through the propagation of action potentials, axons also transport physical material toward the axonal terminal and from the terminal to the cell body. Protein synthesis takes place in the cell body where genetic information is located. Therefore, all proteins and also organelles such as mitochondria that are needed in the axon terminal have to be shipped down the axon with the help of motor proteins. Two motor proteins, kinesin and dynein, move vesicles or organelles along microtubules in the axon.

IntechOpen

Kinesin moves vesicles toward the terminal or away from the center of the neuron (anterograde axonal transport) while dynein moves in the opposite direction, namely from the terminal toward the cell body (retrograde axonal transport).

Glial cells also come in different flavors. Glial cells are increasingly recognized for their physiological functions in the nervous system and have been named "the unsung heroes of the brain" [5]. Certain glial cell types are found only in the peripheral nervous system such as satellite cells or myelin-forming Schwann cells, while others are housed in the central nervous system (brain and spinal cord) such as astrocytes (fibrous and protoplasmic), microglia and myelin-forming oligodendrocytes. Despite these commonly accepted classifications, it should be clear that nerve cells are so varied in their morphology that it has been virtually impossible to adequately classify them based on shape, ultrastructure, neurotransmitter profile, physiology or location. Furthermore, neurons with similar form and function have been described in distant animal taxa that do not share recent phylogenetic relations.

Nerve cells are equipped with cellular machinery that is present in most other cell types such as nucleus, Golgi apparatus, mitochondria, smooth and rough endoplasmic reticulum. Histological staining of nerve cells with dyes such as toluidine blue or cresyl violet (Nissl staining, nucleic acid stain) reveals particularly intense labeling of the nucleolus and Nissl substance in the cytoplasm [6]. Nissl substance refers to free ribosomes in the cytoplasm and bound ribosomes on the ER. This heavy staining pattern is a reflection of the active metabolism and continuous production of peptides and proteins in nerve cells and identifies nerve cells among the most active cells in the body.

3. Excitable cell membranes and channelopathies

Nerve cells and glial cells are compartmentalized by membranes that are built by lipids and proteins. These lipids and proteins are key elements for the unique functional role each neuron plays in the neural circuit and for the intracellular activities that occur in axons and dendrites distant from the cell nucleus. During development, axonal guidance and remodeling of dendritic spines are shaped in response to signal input at local membrane compartments which is communicated to the cell interior through specific receptors and channels. The inside and outside of the cellular membranes are different from each other, such that an asymmetric distribution of lipids and proteins between cytoplasmic and exoplasmic leaflets allows for an unequal division of labor [1]. Lipids are critically relevant for the structure and function of the nervous system. Membrane lipids are the main component of the myelin that ensheathes axons both in the central and peripheral nervous system. Furthermore, at the connections between nerve cells, the synapses, membranes have unique lipid compositions. The synapse is equipped with a synaptic machinery of vesicles and proteins that contribute to the specialized properties of these membrane compartments and to the plastic changes in synaptic transmission from pre- to postsynaptic neurons (synaptic plasticity) [7–9]. Lipid intermediates and lipid modification play roles in signaling pathways related to cell differentiation and in modulating the activity of trophic factors and receptors [1].

Nerve cells are excitable cells with unique properties in transferring information. In order to do so, the membranes of nerve cells are equipped with highly selective pores or ion channels for sodium, potassium, calcium and chloride ions. These channels are critical for membrane excitation and propagation of action potentials. Ion channels are responsive to changes in voltage (voltage gated channels), binding of a chemical (ligand gated channels) or mechanical perturbation.

Channelopathies, disorders of ion channels, are resulting from disturbed ion channel function due to problems with ion channel subunits or regulation of the ion channels [10]. The rapidly growing field of channelopathies started with the discovery of voltage gated channelopathies that result in inherited muscle disease due to mutations in a subunit of the sodium channel or a mutation in a gene coding for a chloride channel in skeletal muscle [10]. Channelopathies have also been identified for ligand gated ion channels due to mutations of a subunit of the glycine receptor or a subunit of the nicotinic acetylcholine receptor [11, 12]. The underlying reasons for channelopathies can be traced back to either inherited causes (congenital, resulting from one or more mutations in the genes encoding the ion channel) or acquired causes such as toxins and autoimmune attack on an ion channel.

4. Neurotransmitters and neuropeptides

The best known neurochemicals are neurotransmitters and neuropeptides since they modulate brain function [1–4]. One set of neurotransmitters is formed by common amino acids such as glutamate, gamma-aminobutyric acid (GABA) and glycine. These amino acids have a number of functions throughout the body. In nerve terminals of neurons, they are packaged and stored in secretory or synaptic vesicles, so they can be released by exocytosis in a calcium dependent manner. The vesicular membrane is recycled, i.e., endocytosed, for future synaptic release cycles. Glutamate is the most prominent excitatory neurotransmitter. It is released at excitatory synapses, and evokes membrane potential depolarization and, possibly, firing of action potentials in the connected postsynaptic cell. In contrast, GABA is the best known inhibitory neurotransmitter. Its action results in reducing neuronal excitability. Glycine is another inhibitory neurotransmitter found in the spinal cord, brainstem and retina. The monoamines form an important group of neurotransmitters involved in regulation of emotion, arousal, some forms of memory as well as sensory processing [1–4, 13, 14]. Because of their functional roles, drugs are used to regulate their effects in patients with psychiatric as well as neurological disorders [15]. As their name implies, monoamines contain an amino group connected to an aromatic ring by a two-carbon chain. The enzymes monoamine oxidases terminate the action of monoamines. Histamine, serotonin, dopamine, epinephrine (adrenaline), norepinephrine (noradrenaline) are monoamines. The latter three are also grouped together as catecholamines because they contain a catechol group. Trace amines such as octopamine, tryptamine, tyramine, phenethylamine and others, have been identified as neurotransmitters. Neuropeptides include compounds such as oxytocin, substance P, somatostatin, opioid peptides, cocaine and amphetamine regulated transcript (CART), glucagon, orexin, dynorphin, endorphin, enkephalin, neuropeptide Y, neuropeptide S, and others. Nitric oxide, hydrogen sulfide and carbon monoxide act as gaseous neurotransmitters [16]. These neurotransmitters are synthesized de novo in nerve cells and because of their chemical nature are able to rapidly diffuse through the plasma membrane to act on neighboring cells. Acetylcholine is released in the autonomic nervous system and also from motor neurons at the neuromuscular junction to evoke skeletal muscle contraction. Chemically, acetylcholine is an ester of acetic acid and choline. Endogenously produced cannabinoids (endocannabinoids) such as anandamide differ from the above mentioned neurotransmitters because they are formed from membrane lipids and are essentially lipids. They can be rapidly synthesized on demand from the cell membrane and released nonsynaptically and not from synaptic vesicles as the classic neurotransmitters, reviewed in [9, 17, 18]. Endocannabinoids bind to cannabinoid receptors on presynaptic neurons to regulate presynaptic neurotransmitter release. Therefore, endocannabinoids together with the gaseous neurotransmitters are unusual neurotransmitters [17, 19, 20]. One key distinction of these novel neurotransmitters is the fact that they act as retrograde messengers at synapses and presynaptically regulate either glutamatergic or GABAergic synapses to alter release-probability in synaptic plasticity. Gaseous neurotransmitters and endocannabinoids have been shown to have a functional role in experience-dependent activity and mediate a variety of forms of short- and long-term synaptic plasticity [21–24].

5. Factors that influence neurochemistry

What are some of the factors that affect the chemistry of the nervous system? Factors that modify neurochemistry include sensory stimuli, environmental signals such as recreational drugs, pharmaceuticals and toxins, and bodily changes such as aging and disease. Listed below, and described in more detail, are examples of some such factors known to influence neurochemistry. It is important to realize that this list is not exhaustive, and that in theory almost any external stimulus or internal state could influence neurochemistry.

5.1 Sleep

Sleep is controlled by circadian rhythms, which have a neurochemical (and oscillatory epigenetic) basis. During waking, several brain structures participate, namely the basal forebrain, posterior and lateral hypothalamus, and nuclei in the tegmentum and pons. Neurotransmitters that act as significant wakefulness factors are acetylcholine and monoamines, glutamate and hypocretin/orexin. Conversely, the preoptic/anterior hypothalamic area regulates active sleep mechanisms, and sleep is promoted by GABA and peptide factors, including growth hormone-releasing hormone, cytokines, and prolactin [25]. Adenosine is a significant homeostatic factor acting in basal forebrain and preoptic areas via A1 and A2A receptors. Lack of sleep increases inducible nitric oxide synthase in the basal forebrain, which causes adenosine release and recovery sleep. Also, many genes have been found differentially expressed in wakefulness versus sleep, and they relate to neural transmission, energy metabolism, stress protection, and synaptic plasticity [25].

5.2 Exercise

There has recently been a large amount of research into the neurochemical changes that occur during and after exercise, finding that it stimulates the increase of many chemicals, namely lactate, cortisol, neurotrophins, including BDNF, VEGF and IGF-1, neurotransmitters, including dopamine, serotonin, norepinephrine, GABA, acetylcholine, and glutamate, and neuromodulators, including endocannabinoids and endogenous opioids [26]. However, it should be noted that many of these alterations have been demonstrated only peripherally, and gaps still exist in our knowledge as to exactly where these changes occur in the brain. Therefore, further work is needed to link the exercise-induced changes in peripheral levels to central levels, and to understand how these chemicals are involved in the exercise-induced changes in cognition, mood, and so forth [26].

5.3 Diet

The scientific field concerned with the effects various contents of the diet such as macronutrients, and micronutrients such as minerals, vitamins, dietary supplements, and food additives have on neurochemistry is called "nutritional neuroscience." Recent research on nutrition and its effect on the brain show that it is involved in almost every aspect of neurological function, modulating neurotrophic factors, neural pathways, neurogenesis, and neuroplasticity [27]. This is not surprising when we consider that the brain consumes a very large amount of energy relative to the rest of the body. Specifically, the human brain is approximately 2% of the body mass but uses up to 25% of the energy input. Therefore, mechanisms involved in the transfer of energy from foods to neurons are likely to be essential to the control of brain function. Furthermore, insufficient intake of certain vitamins and other cofactors, or the consequences of metabolic disorders such as diabetes, affect cognition by altering processes in the body that are associated with the management of energy and synthesis of neurotrophic and neuroendocrine factors (i.e., BDNF and IGF-1) as well as neurotransmitter in neurons, which can subsequently affect neurotransmission, synaptic plasticity, and cell survival [27].

5.4 Stress

Stress has been defined as a brain-body reaction to stimuli from the environment or from internal states that are interpreted by the body as disrupted homeostasis [28]. The response to such stress involves both the activity of different neurotransmitters in the limbic system, and the response of neurons there to other chemicals and hormones, mainly glucocorticoids, released from the adrenal cortex. Thus, body-brain integration probably plays a major role in the stress response [28]. Specifically, acute stress is correlated with alterations of neurotransmitters such as dopamine, acetylcholine, GABA and glutamate in areas of the brain associated with the regulation of stress responses. These areas include the prefrontal cortex, amygdala, nucleus accumbens, and hippocampus. Glucocorticoids also play an important role, and interact with several neurotransmitters in those same areas of the brain. Also, the actions of neuromodulators released from peripheral organs such as the liver (IGF-1), pancreas (insulin), or gonads (estrogens) play a role [28]. A permanent increase in the baseline levels of glucocorticoids arising from a stressful lifestyle could exacerbate neuronal damage that occurs in the above areas of the brain during aging. Conversely, stress reduction may have an anti-aging effect [29].

5.5 Meditation

One way to counteract stress is through practices such as meditation and yoga. These techniques have recently received increased attention due to the accumulation of research showing both direct and indirect benefits [30]. Based on studies conducted so far, it has been found that the practice of meditation influences the levels of neurotransmitters such as GABA, serotonin, dopamine, and norepinephrine, in a way that positively affects psychological disorders such as anxiety. Also, by reducing baseline levels of stress hormones and neurotransmitters, meditation may act as a form of preventative medicine [30].

5.6 Alcohol

Alcohol has effects on many neurotransmitters in the brain. Its major effect is to stimulate the release of GABA, and it acts principally at the GABAA receptors, and thereby has sedative effects [31]. It also inhibits postsynaptic NMDA excitatory glutamate receptors, and this inhibition further contributes to the sedation.

However, alcohol also has euphoric effects, and these are more related to increases in dopamine. The effects on dopamine are also thought to be involved in alcohol craving and relapse. In addition, alcohol alters opioid receptors and can lead to a release of β-endorphins. Additional important effects include increased serotonin and decreased nicotinic acetylcholine receptors [31].

5.7 Recreational drugs

Drugs can alter the regular functions of neurochemicals, inhibit the way they are supposed to act, or disrupt their communication [32]. At first, pleasure is usually increased, but cognitive ability and rationality are decreased. Psychomotor stimulant drugs like amphetamines, methamphetamine, and cocaine cause an overproduction of neurotransmitters, principally the monoamines dopamine and norepinephrine, and may also prevent them from being reabsorbed, causing an abnormally large amount to be present in synapses, and thereby activate the mesolimbic dopamine system. Drugs like ecstasy (3,4-methalynedioxymethamphetamine) similarly interfere with the transmission of serotonin, and the way it is transported along neural pathways. Other drugs, such as heroin, opioids, and marijuana, mimic endogenous brain chemicals and bind to receptors as agonists, activating the neurons and thus disrupting the natural transmission and production of neurotransmitters [32]. With repeated drug abuse, the brain can be rewired via neuroplasticity as it attempts to maintain chemical homeostasis [33].

5.8 Neurodegenerative diseases and aging

Studies of the neurobiology of aging are beginning to uncover the mechanisms underlying not only the physiology of aging of the brain, but also the mechanisms that make people more vulnerable to cognitive dysfunction and neurodegenerative diseases [29]. Neurotransmission is impaired in age-related disorders, such as Alzheimer's and Parkinson's diseases, which has stimulated investigations into the neurochemistry of the aging human brain. Out of all the neurotransmitter systems studied, age-related changes in the serotonergic, cholinergic, and dopaminergic systems are the most reliably found [34]. The dopamine system in particular, is especially vulnerable to aging [35]. The association of these neurotransmitters with mood, memory, and motor function may contribute to age-associated behavioral changes and predispose older people to age-related diseases. Moreover, age-related neurodegenerative diseases may evolve from the interaction between defects in specific neurochemical mechanisms and other pathophysiologic processes [33].

Acknowledgements

This work was supported in part by grants from the National Science Foundation (NSF IOS-1355034) and the Charles and Mary Latham Trust Fund to TH and from the National Institutes of Health (NIH) to ABC.

Conflict of interest

The authors declare that there is no conflict of interests regarding the publication of this chapter.

DOI: http://dx.doi.org/10.5772/intechopen.89072

Author details

Thomas Heinbockel* and Antonei B. Csoka
Department of Anatomy, Howard University College of Medicine,
Washington, DC, USA

*Address all correspondence to: theinbockel@howard.edu

References

[1] Brady ST, Siegel JG, Albers BW, Price DL. Basic Neurochemistry, Principles of Molecular, Cellular, and Medical Neurobiology. 8th ed. Boston: Elsevier; 2012. DOI: 10.1016/C2009-0-00066-X. ISBN: 978-0-12-374947-5

[2] Purves D, Augustine GJ, Fitzpatrick D, Hall WC, LaMantia AS, White LE. Neuroscience. 5th ed. Sunderland: Sinauer; 2012. ISBN: 978-0-87893-695-3

[3] Kandel ER, Schwartz JH, Jessell TM, Siegelbaum SA, Hudspeth AJ. Principles of Neural Science. 5th ed. New York: McGraw-Hill; 2013. ISBN: 978-0-07-139011-8

[4] Bear M, Connors BW, Paradiso MA. Neuroscience—Exploring the Brain. 4th ed. Philadelphia: Wolters Kluwer; 2016. ISBN: 978-0-7817-7817-6

[5] Young JK. Introduction to Cell Biology. New Jersey: World Scientific Publishing Co. Pte. Ltd.; 2010. ISBN-13: 978-981-4307-31-4

[6] Telser AG, Young JK, Baldwin KM. Elsevier's Integrated Histology. Philadelphia: Mosby Elsevier; 2007. ISBN: 978-0-323-03388-6

[7] Sheng M, Sabatini BL, Südhof TC. The Synapse. Cold Spring Harbor, New York: Cold Spring Harbor Laboratory Press; 2012. 397pp

[8] Citri A, Malenka RC. Synaptic plasticity: Multiple forms, functions, and mechanisms. Neuropsychopharmacology. 2008;**33**:18-41. DOI: 10.1038/sj.npp.1301559

[9] Heinbockel T, editor. Introductory chapter: Mechanisms and function of synaptic plasticity. In: Synaptic Plasticity. Rijeka, Croatia: InTech Publisher; 2017. pp. 3-13. DOI: 10.5772/67891

[10] Rose MR. Dysfunctional ion channels may cause many neurological diseases. BMJ. 1998;**316**(7138):1104-1105. DOI: 10.1136/bmj.316.7138.1104

[11] Shiang R, Ryan SG, Zhu YZ, Hahn AF, O'Connell P, Wasmuth JJ. Mutations in the alpha 1 subunit of the inhibitory glycine receptor cause the dominant neurologic disorder, hyperekplexia. Nature Genetics. 1993;**5**:351-358

[12] Steinlein OK, Mulley JC, Propping P, Wallace RH, Phillips HA, Scheffer IE, et al. A missense mutation in the neuronal nicotinic acetylcholine receptor alpha 4 subunit is associated with autosomal dominant nocturnal frontal lobe epilepsy. Nature Genetics. 1995;**11**:201-203

[13] Bloom FE. The functional significance of neurotransmitter diversity. The American Journal of Physiology. 1984;**246**(3 Pt 1): C184-C194

[14] Jacob SN, Nienborg H. Monoaminergic neuromodulation of sensory processing. Front Neural Circuits. 2018;**12**:51. DOI: 10.3389/fncir.2018.00051. eCollection 2018

[15] Kurian MA, Gissen P, Smith M, Heales SJR, Clayton PT. The monoamine neurotransmitter disorders: An expanding range of neurological syndromes. The Lancet Neurology. 2011;**10**(8):721-733. DOI: 10.1016/S1474-4422(11)70141-7

[16] Haley JE. Gases as neurotransmitters. Essays in Biochemistry. 1998;**33**:79-91

[17] Heinbockel T, editor. Chapter 6: Neurochemical communication: The case of endocannabinoids. In: Neurochemistry. Rijeka, Croatia: InTech Open Access Publisher; 2014. pp. 179-198. ISBN: 978-953-51-1237-2

[18] Heinbockel T, Wang ZJ, Brown EA, Austin PT. Endocannabinoid signaling in neural circuits of the olfactory and limbic system 2. In: Meccariello R, Chianese R, editors. Cannabinoids in Health and Disease. Rijeka, Croatia: InTech Publisher; 2016. pp. 11-37. ISBN: 978-953-51-2429-0

[19] Barañano DE, Ferris CD, Snyder SH. Atypical neural messengers. Trends in Neurosciences. 2001;**24**:99-106

[20] Boehning D, Snyder SH. Novel neural modulators. Annual Review of Neuroscience. 2003;**26**:105-131

[21] Hardingham N, Dachtler J, Fox K. The role of nitric oxide in pre-synaptic plasticity and homeostasis. Frontiers in Cellular Neuroscience. 2013;**31**(7):190

[22] Cachope R. Functional diversity on synaptic plasticity mediated by endocannabinoids. Philosophical Transactions of the Royal Society of London. Series B, Biological Sciences. 2012;**367**:3242-3253

[23] Castillo PE, Younts TJ, Chávez AE, Hashimotodani Y. Endocannabinoid signaling and synaptic function. Neuron. 2012;**76**:70-81

[24] Katona I, Freund TF. Multiple functions of endocannabinoid signaling in the brain. Annual Review of Neuroscience. 2012;**35**:529-558

[25] Stenberg D. Neuroanatomy and neurochemistry of sleep. Cellular and Molecular Life Sciences. 2007;**64**:1187-1204

[26] Basso JC, Suzuki WA. The effects of acute exercise on mood, cognition, neurophysiology, and neurochemical pathways: A review. Brain Plasticity. 2017;**28**(2):127-152

[27] Dauncey MJ. New insights into nutrition and cognitive neuroscience. The Proceedings of the Nutrition Society. 2009;**68**:408-415

[28] Mora F, Segovia G, Del Arco A, de Blas M, Garrido P. Stress, neurotransmitters, corticosterone and body-brain integration. Brain Research. 2012;**1476**:71-85

[29] Mora F. Successful brain aging: Plasticity, environmental enrichment, and lifestyle. Dialogues in Clinical Neuroscience. 2013;**15**:45-52

[30] Krishnakumar D, Hamblin MR, Lakshmanan S. Meditation and yoga can modulate brain mechanisms that affect behavior and anxiety—A modern scientific perspective. Ancient Science. 2015;**2**:13-19

[31] Banerjee N. Neurotransmitters in alcoholism: A review of neurobiological and genetic studies. Indian Journal of Human Genetics. 2014;**20**:20-31

[32] Korpi ER, den Hollander B, Farooq U, Vashchinkina E, Rajkumar R, Nutt DJ, et al. Mechanisms of action and persistent neuroplasticity by drugs of abuse. Pharmacological Reviews. 2015;**67**:872-1004

[33] Leshner AI, Koob GF. Drugs of abuse and the brain. Proceedings of the Association of American Physicians. 1999;**111**:99-108

[34] Strong R. Neurochemical changes in the aging human brain: Implications for behavioral impairment and neurodegenerative disease. Geriatrics. 1998;**53**(Suppl 1):S9-S12

[35] Dreher JC, Meyer-Lindenberg A, Kohn P, Berman KF. Age-related changes in midbrain dopaminergic regulation of the human reward system. Proceedings of the National Academy of Sciences of the United States of America. 2008;**105**:15106-15111

Chapter 2

Synaptic Transmission and Amino Acid Neurotransmitters

Manorama Patri

Abstract

Amino acids are the most abundant neurotransmitters in the brain. Neurotransmitters are synthesized and stored in presynaptic terminals, released from terminals upon stimulation with specific receptors on the postsynaptic cells. Chemical and electrical synapses are specialized biological structures found in the nervous system; they connect neurons together and transmit signals across the neurons. The process of synaptic transmission generates or inhibits electrical impulses in a network of neurons for the processing of information. Glutamate is the primary excitatory neurotransmitter in the brain, while GABA is the principal inhibitory neurotransmitter. The balance of glutamatergic and GABAergic tone is crucial to normal neurologic function. Through synaptic transmission, this information is communicated from the presynaptic cell to the postsynaptic cell. Amino acid neurotransmitters primarily glutamic acid, GABA, aspartic acid, and glycine are single amino acid residues released from presynaptic nerve terminals in response to an action potential and cross the synaptic cleft to bind with specific receptor on the postsynaptic membrane. The integral role of amino acid neurotransmitters is important on the normal functioning of the brain. The presynaptic and postsynaptic events in chemical synapses are subject to use dependent and highly regulated as per the changes in synaptic neurotransmitter release and function.

Keywords: synapse, neurotransmitter, receptor, glutamate, GABA, glycine, aspartate

1. Introduction

The nervous system is composed of billions of specialized cells called neurons. Neurons are the cells of chemical communication in the brain. In its most basic form, a neuron has two ends (although either can have multiple branches): an axon and a dendrite (**Figure 1**). Efficient communication between neuronal cells is a crucial process for the normal functioning of the central and peripheral nervous system. Neurotransmitters are chemical substances that act as the mediator for the transmission of nerve impulses from one neuron to another neuron through synapses. Neurotransmitters are stored in the axon (or presynaptic neuron) in little packages called synaptic vesicles. The release of neurotransmitter is triggered by the arrival of nerve impulse (or action potential). Synapses are specialized junctions through which cells of the nervous system signal to one another and to non-neuronal cells such as muscles or glands. The process by which the information is communicated through synapse is called synaptic transmission [1, 2].

The neurotransmitters are stored in the vesicles within the presynaptic nerve terminal at the synaptic membrane of one nerve cell and released into the synaptic cleft in response to nerve impulses [2]. The secreted neurotransmitters can then act on receptors on the membrane of the postsynaptic neuron through a gap called synaptic gap (0.02 micron). The number of synaptic contacts of an average neuron is approximately 10,000. Thus, there are 3–5 × 10^{15} synapses in the human brain. There are two types of synapses, electrical and chemical synapses, but chemical synapses (**Figure 2**) far outnumber electrical ones. Electric synapses are gap junction. A gap junction is a junction between neurons that allows different molecules and ions to pass freely between cells. The junction connects the cytoplasm of cells. A gap junction is composed of connexons (each connexon is composed of six connexin proteins) which connect across the intercellular space. Neurons connected by gap junctions sometimes act as though they were equivalent to one large neuron with many output pathways, all of which fire synchronously.

Synapses are made on all regions of a receiving nerve cell and can be classified on the basis where they are located. On spiny dendrites of a nerve cell, each spine is the target of an axon terminal and comprises the postsynaptic component of a single synapse. Synapses between axons and dendrites are called axodendritic. Particularly powerful synapses are made between axons of one neuron and cell body of another postsynaptic cell. These are called axosomatic synapses. Synapses between axon terminals and axons of postsynaptic neurons are said to be axo-axonal.

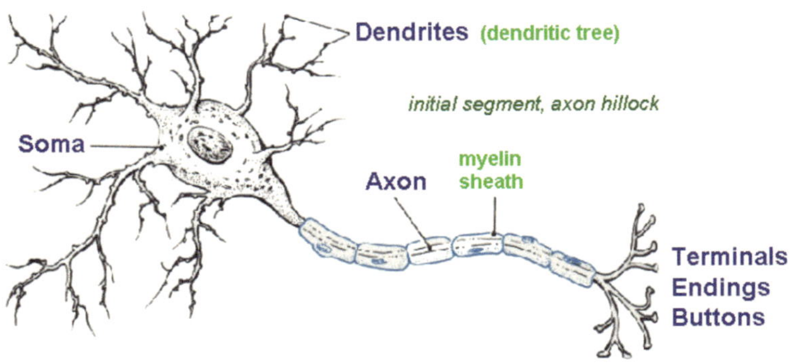

Figure 1.
Structure of neuron.

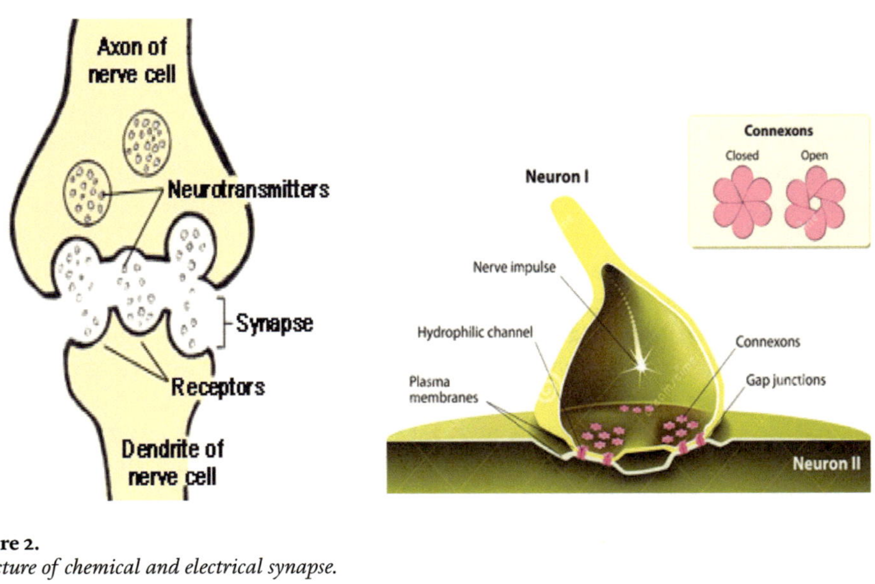

Figure 2.
Structure of chemical and electrical synapse.

Substances that act as neurotransmitters can be categorized into different groups. The three major categories of substances that act as neurotransmitters are:

1. Amino acids: The neurotransmitters of this group are involved in fast synaptic transmission and are inhibitory and excitatory in action (primarily glutamic acid, GABA, aspartic acid, and glycine).

2. Amines: Amines are the modified amino acids such as biogenic amines, e.g., catecholamines. The neurotransmitters of this group involve in slow synaptic transmission and are inhibitory and excitatory in action (noradrenaline, adrenaline, dopamine, serotonin, and histamine).

3. Others: The one which do not fit in any of these categories (acetyl choline and nitric oxide). Amino acids are among the most abundant of all neurotransmitters present within the central nervous system (CNS).

Several amino acids have been implicated as neurotransmitters in the CNS, including GABA, glutamic acid, glycine, and aspartic acid [3]. Some (like glutamate) are excitatory, whereas others (like GABA) are primarily inhibitory. Aspartate is closely related to glutamate, and the two amino acids are often are found together at axon terminals. Neurons synthesize glutamate and aspartate and are independent of dietary supply.

1.1 Function of amino acid neurotransmitter

The amino acid neurotransmitters are common neurotransmitters in the central nervous system. Glycine, glutamate, and GABA are classed under amino acid neurotransmitter. The two amino acids functioning as excitatory neurotransmitter are glutamate and aspartate. GABA acts as a brake to the excitatory neurotransmitters, and thus when it is abnormally low, this can lead to anxiety, and glutamate usually ensures homeostasis with the effects of GABA [4]. Several related amino acids, like homocysteic acid and N-acetylaspartylglutamate, may also serve a neurotransmitter function. Neurotransmitters can be classified as either excitatory or inhibitory. Excitatory neurotransmitters function to activate the receptors on the postsynaptic membrane and enhance the effects of action potential, while inhibitory neurotransmitter functions in a reverse mechanism. If the electrical impulses transmitted inward toward the cell body are large enough, they will generate an action potential.

The action potentials are caused by an exchange of ions across the neuron membrane; a stimulus first causes sodium channels to open, because there are many more sodium ions on the outside, and the inside of the neuron is negative relative to the outside; sodium ions rush into the neuron. Since sodium has a positive charge, the neuron becomes more positive and becomes depolarized. It takes longer for potassium channels to open; when they do open, potassium rushes out of the cell, reversing the depolarization. Also at about this time, sodium channels start to close; this causes the action potential to go back toward −70 mv (a repolarization). The action potential actually goes past (overshoots) −70 mv (a hyperpolarization) because the potassium channels stay open a bit too long. Gradually, the ion concentrations go back to resting levels, and the cell returns to −70 mv.

The action potential is produced by an influx of calcium ions through voltage-dependent calcium-selective ion channels. Calcium ions then trigger a biochemical cascade which results in neurotransmitter vesicles fusing with the presynaptic membrane and releasing their contents to the synaptic cleft. Receptors on the opposite side of the synaptic gap bind neurotransmitter molecules and respond by opening nearby ion channels in the postsynaptic cell membrane, causing ions to rush in or out and changing the local transmembrane potential of the cell. The resulting change in voltage is called a postsynaptic potential. The result is excitatory, in the case of depolarizing currents, or inhibitory in the case of hyperpolarizing currents resulting in EPSP or IPSP, respectively (**Figure 3**).

Whether a synapse is excitatory or inhibitory depends on what type(s) of ion channel conduct the postsynaptic current, which in turn is a function of the type of receptors and neurotransmitter employed at the synapse. Neurotransmitters may have excitatory effects if they drive a cell's membrane to the threshold of an action potential (**Figure 4**).

The resting potential of a neuron tells about what happens when a neuron is at rest. An action potential occurs when a neuron sends information down an axon, away from the cell body. The action potential is an explosion of electrical activity that is created by a depolarizing current. This means that a stimulus causes the resting potential to move toward 0 mv.

1. When the depolarization near the axon hillock reaches about −55 mv as a result of summation of EPSPs, a neuron will fire an action potential. This is the threshold. If the neuron does not reach this critical threshold level, then no action potential will fire.

2. Also, when the threshold level is reached, an action potential of a fixed sized will always fire for any given neuron; the size of the action potential is always the same.

There are no big or small action potentials in one nerve cell. All action potentials are the same in size in a particular neuron type (it can differ between different types of neurons). Therefore, either the neuron does not reach the threshold or a full action potential is fired—this is the "all or none" principle.

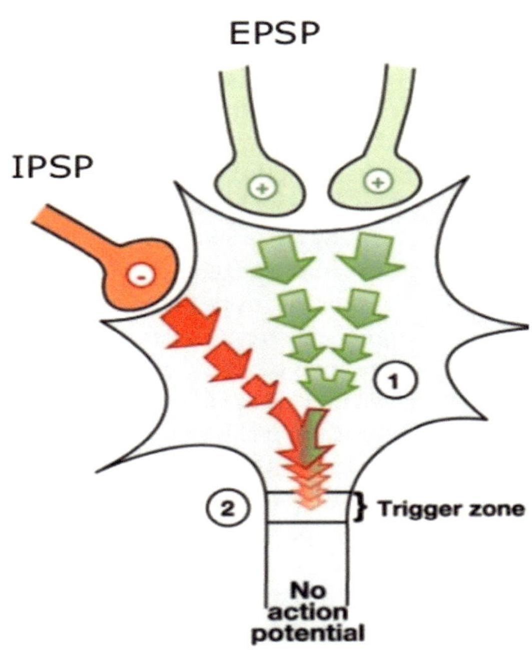

Figure 3.
EPSP and IPSP on a neuron.

DOI: http://dx.doi.org/10.5772/intechopen.82121

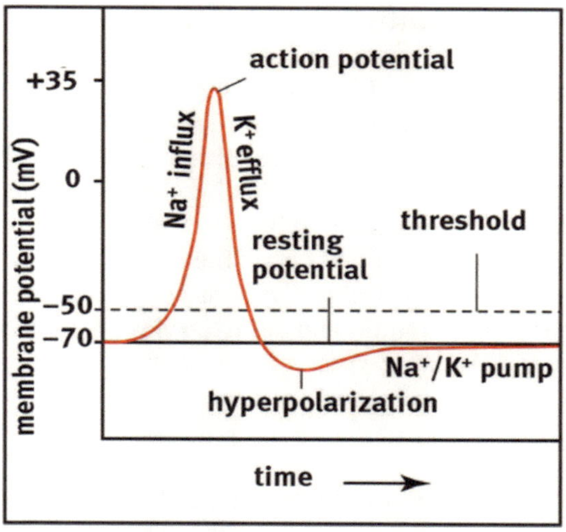

Figure 4.
Action potential.

A neuron encodes the intensity of a stimulus in the frequency of firing and not in the size of a single impulse. Neurotransmitters may have inhibitory effects if they help to drive the membrane away from threshold. An excitatory postsynaptic potential (EPSP) is a summation of signals that brings the membrane closer to the threshold (depolarizing effect). An inhibitory postsynaptic potential (IPSP) drives the membrane away from threshold by a hyperpolarizing effect.

1.1.1 Excitatory neurotransmitters

An excitatory postsynaptic potential (EPSP) is a temporary increase in postsynaptic membrane potential within dendrites or cell bodies caused by the flow of sodium ions into the postsynaptic cell. EPSPs are additive. Larger EPSPs result in greater membrane depolarization and thus increase the likelihood that the postsynaptic cell reaches the threshold for firing an action potential. When an active presynaptic cell releases neurotransmitters into the synapse, some of them bind to receptors on the postsynaptic cell. Many of these receptors contain an ion channel capable of passing positively charged ions either into or out of the cell. At excitatory synapses, the ion channel typically allows sodium into the cell, generating an excitatory postsynaptic current.

1.1.2 Inhibitory neurotransmitters

GABA and glycine are inhibitory, both instead of depolarizing the postsynaptic membrane and producing an EPSP; they hyperpolarize the postsynaptic membrane and produce IPSP. IPSP is the change in membrane voltage of a postsynaptic neuron which results from synaptic activation of inhibitory neurotransmitter receptors. The most common inhibitory neurotransmitters in the nervous system are γ-aminobutyric acid (GABA) and glycine. At a typical inhibitory synapse, the postsynaptic neural membrane permeability increases for K^+ ions and Cl^- ions but not for Na^+ ions.

This generally causes an influx of chloride ions and efflux of K^+ ions, thereby bringing the membrane potential closer to the equilibrium potential of these ions.

2. Amino acid neurotransmitters

Amino acid transmitters provide the majority of excitatory and inhibitory neurotransmission in the nervous system. Amino acids used for synaptic transmission are compartmentalized (e.g., glutamate, compartmentalized from metabolic glutamate used for protein synthesis by packaging the transmitter into synaptic vesicles for subsequent Ca^{2+}-dependent release). Amino acid neurotransmitters are all products of intermediary metabolism with the exception of GABA. Unlike all the other amino acid neurotransmitters, GABA is not used in protein synthesis and is produced by an enzyme (glutamic acid decarboxylase; GAD) uniquely located in neurons. Antibodies to GAD can be used to identify neurons that release GABA.

2.1 Glutamate

Glutamate is used at the great majority of fast excitatory synapses in the brain and spinal cord. Glutamatergic neurons are particularly prominent in the cerebral cortex. They project to a variety of subcortical structures like the hippocampus, the basolateral complex of the amygdala, the substantia nigra, the nucleus accumbens, the superior colliculus, the caudate nucleus (nucleus ruber), and the pons. At glutamatergic synapses, NMDA receptors (NMDARs) are localized with other ionotropic glutamate receptors [AMPA receptors (AMPARs) and kainate receptors] and with metabotropic glutamate receptors. Glutamate receptors are necessary for neuronal development, synaptic plasticity, excitotoxicity, pain perception, and learning and memory [5]. Among these EPSP-producing glutamate receptors, which could occur as homomeric or heteromeric structures, are classified according to the binding of the most common agonist [6].

Four subtypes can be distinguished, out of which three are ionotropic receptors and one metabotropic receptor, activated by quisqualate. These are named according to the molecules (other than glutamate) that they bind and include:

1. NMDA receptors (named for N-methyl-D-aspartate)

2. AMPA receptors (α-amino-3-hydroxy-5-methyl-4-isoxazolepropionate)

3. Kainate receptors

4. Receptors which are activated by quisqualate

2.1.1 NMDA receptors

NMDA receptor is very important for controlling developmental synaptic plasticity and learning and memory function. NMDARs have critical roles in excitatory synaptic transmission, plasticity, and excitotoxicity in the CNS (**Figure 5**). The NR1 subunit is evenly expressed in most of the brain, but the NR2 subunit (NR2A, NR2B, NR2C, and NR2D) shows distinct regional distributions [6, 7]. NMDA receptors show three specific properties by which they differ from other types of ionotropic receptors:

a. NMDA receptor ion channel is subjected to voltage-dependent block by the extracellular Mg^{2+} ion.

b. They display a high permeability to Ca^{2+} ions. Ca^{2+} influx through NMDA receptor channel leads to a cascade of intracellular events triggering long-term potentiation (LTP) and long-term depression (LTD) of synaptic currents.

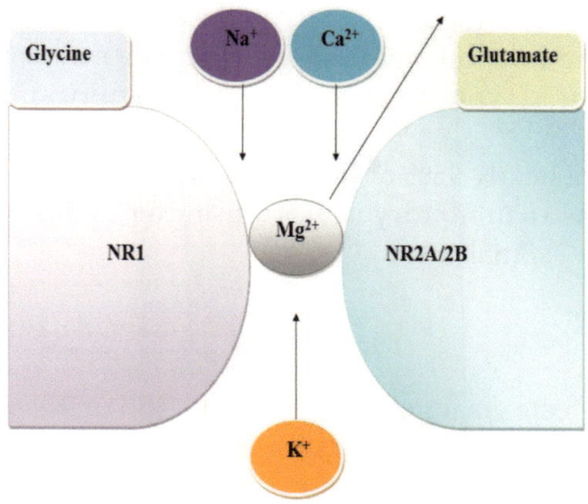

Figure 5.
NMDA receptor.

c. The response of NMDA receptor to neurotransmitter like glutamate and glycine under physiological conditions is modified by certain extracellular molecules like H^+, Zn^{2+}, and polyamines. Most of the NMDA receptors function only in heteromeric assemblies, composed of two NR1 and two NR2 subunits.

Glutamate binds to the S1 and S2 regions of NR2 subunit, whereas glycine binds to the S1 and S2 regions of NR1 subunit. Individual NR1 or NR2 subunits contain an extracellular N terminus which forms S1, an intracellular C terminus, and an extracellular loop between M3 and M4 that constitutes S2. The channel lining domain is formed by a reentrant pore loop called as M2 loop that enters the channel from the cytoplasmic side and forms a narrow constriction at that channel. The critical asparagine residue located within M2 loop determines the selectivity of NMDAR channel for Mg^{2+} block and Ca^{2+} permeability.

The function of NMDA receptors is totally dependent upon AMPA receptors. In the absence of AMPA, NMDA is initially expressed, and it forms the silent synapse. The NMDA receptors are not activated unless the postsynaptic region is depolarized by AMPA receptors.

AMPA receptors are ionotropic and belong to the group of non-NMDA receptors and associated with a cation-selective ion channel which is permeable for monovalent cations, like Na^+ and K^+. Under certain combinatorial conditions of the receptor subunits, it also becomes permeable to Ca^{2+}.

Kainate receptors can be activated by kainite and glutamate. Like AMPA receptors, the kainite receptors are associated with an ionic channel which is permeable for the monovalent cations Na^+ K^+ and for Ca^{2+}. These receptors are mainly involved in modulating the release of excitatory amino acids and additional neurotransmitters or neuromodulators.

The metabotropic receptors are activated by glutamate and quisqualate and resistant to activation by NMDA, AMPA, or kainate.

2.2 GABA

GABA is the most ubiquitous inhibitory neurotransmitter in the brain. GABA was discovered in 1883, and its inhibitory function was described in the late 1950s by Bazemore et al. [8]. It was the first amino acid to be established as a neurotransmitter in vertebrate and invertebrate nervous systems. GABA is synthesized in nervous tissue exclusively from glutamate by the alpha decarboxylation of glutamic acid in the presence of glutamic acid decarboxylase (GAD). The apparent prominent role of GAD in modulation of GABA levels becomes obvious under pathological conditions, where GAD concentration can differ significantly from normal levels.

Striatum contained nearly 95% of the cells which are GABAergic. GABA is also suspected to operate as an inhibitory neurotransmitter in the cerebral cortex, lateral vestibular nucleus, and spinal cord.

2.2.1 GABA receptors

GABA exerts its effects via ionotropic ($GABA_A$) and metabotropic ($GABA_B$) receptors. $GABA_A$ receptors show a ubiquitous distribution throughout the CNS and have been identified on both neuron and glia. GABA can act on both rapid and slow inhibitory receptors (the $GABA_A$ and $GABA_B$), respectively. $GABA_A$ receptors are chloride channels that in response to GABA binding increases chloride influx into the neuron. The agonist of these receptors includes GABA and muscimol. The $GABA_B$ receptors are potassium channels that when activated by GABA leads to potassium efflux from the cell. $GABA_A$ receptors are ionotropic receptors leading to increased Cl^- ion conductance, whereas $GABA_B$ receptors are metabotropic receptors which are coupled to G proteins and thereby indirectly alter membrane ion permeability and neuronal excitability [4].

2.3 Glycine

Glycine is the simplest of amino acids, consisting of an amino group and a carboxyl (acidic) group attached to a carbon atom. In mammals, glycine belongs to the nonessential amino acids [9]. Until the early 1960s, glycine was of minor importance in synaptic transmission because of its simple structure and its ubiquitous distribution as a member of protein and nucleotide metabolism. Glycine's function is a potent neurotransmitter in the spinal cord and brain. Glycine is a constituent of glutathione, an antioxidant tripeptide found in high concentrations in intestinal epithelial cells. The availability of glycine has the potential to control the cellular levels of glutathione in enterocytes. This amino acid functions as an excitatory transmitter during embryonic development and is an essential coagonist at glutamatergic synapses containing the NMDA subtype of glutamate receptors. Hydroxymethyl transferase converts the amino acid serine to glycine. More recently, glycine has been found to play a role in the functional modulation of NMDA receptors.

2.3.1 Glycine receptor

Glycine receptors are ligand-gated ion channels that increase Cl^- influx. Glycine molecules may be taken back into the presynaptic cell by two high-affinity glycine transporters (Glyt-1 and Glyt-2). Glyt-1 is found primarily in glial cells, whereas Glty-2 is found primarily in neuronal cells. The transport of glycine via Glyt-1 is coupled to the movement of Na^+ and Cl^-, with a Na^+:Cl^-:glycine stoichiometry of 2:1:1.

The glycine receptor GlyR belongs to the superfamily of ligand-gated ion channels, like $GABA_A$, and is primarily found in the ventral spinal cord. Strychnine is a glycine antagonist which can bind to the glycine receptor without opening the chloride ion channel (i.e., it inhibits inhibition). GlyR is a strychnine-sensitive glycoprotein which is composed of five subunits. The receptor has a pentameric structure with three ligand-binding α subunits and two β subunits forming an ion channel. This heterogenicity is responsible for the distinct pharmaceutical and functional properties displayed by the various receptor configurations that are differentially expressed and assembled during development [10].

The glycine receptor is presently considered to form a complex consisting of a glycine recognition site and an associated chloride channel. Hyperekplexia, or startle disease, is a rare neurological disorder characterized by an exaggerated response to unexpected stimuli. The response is typically accompanied by a transient but complete muscular rigidity (stiff baby syndrome).

2.4 Aspartate

Glutamate and aspartate are nonessential amino acids that do not cross the blood-brain barrier and, therefore, are synthesized from glucose and a variety of other precursors. The synthetic and metabolic enzymes for glutamate and aspartate have been localized to the two main compartments of the brain, neurons and glial cells. Aspartate is the most abundant excitatory neurotransmitter in the CNS. Like glycine, aspartate is primarily localized to the ventral spinal cord. Like glycine, aspartate opens an ion channel and is inactivated by reabsorption into the presynaptic membrane. Unlike glycine, however, aspartate is an excitatory neurotransmitter, which increases the likelihood of depolarization in the postsynaptic membrane [9, 10]. Aspartate is a highly selective agonist for NMDAR-type glutamate receptors and does not activate AMPA-type glutamate receptors. Hence, synapses only releasing aspartate should therefore generate only NMDAR currents despite a full postsynaptic complement of AMPARs [11].

Aspartate and glycine form an excitatory/inhibitory pair in the ventral spinal cord comparable to the excitatory/inhibitory pair formed by glutamate and GABA in the brain. Interestingly, the two excitatory amino acids, glutamic acid and aspartic acid, are the two acidic amino acids found in proteins, insofar as both have two carboxyl groups rather than one. Thus, variation in the vesicular content of glutamate and aspartate might have a profound effect on the relative contribution of NMDARs and AMPARs to synaptic transmission [12, 13].

3. Conclusion

Neurotransmitters are the brain chemicals that communicate information throughout our brain and body. They relay signals between neurons. Amino acid neurotransmitters can be subdivided into the excitatory amino acids aspartate and glutamate and the inhibitory amino acids GABA and glycine. Common inhibitory neurotransmitters such as GABA and glycine calm the brain and help create balance, whereas excitatory neurotransmitters such as glutamate and aspartate stimulate the brain.

Acknowledgements

The author is thankful to the support by funding from the Project DAE-BRNS, Mumbai, No. 37(1)14/27/2015/ BRNS and DRDO, New Delhi, No. O/o DG (TM)/81/48222/LSRB-294/PEE&BS/2017.

Conflict of interest

The authors declare that they have no conflict of interest.

Author details

Manorama Patri
Neurobiology Laboratory, Department of Zoology, School of Life Sciences, Ravenshaw University, Cuttack, Odisha, India

*Address all correspondence to: mpatri@ravenshawuniversity.ac.in

References

[1] Lodish H, Berk A, Zipursky SL. Molecular Cell Biology: Section 21.4 Neurotransmitters, Synapses, and Impulse Transmission. 4th ed. New York: W. H. Freeman; 2000

[2] Ayano G. Common Neurotransmitters: Criteria for neurotransmitters, key locations, classifications and functions. Advances in Psychology and Neuroscience. 2016;**4**(6):91-95

[3] Oliver VB, Halbach DR. Neurotransmitters and Neuromodulators: Handbook of Receptors and Biological Effects. 2nd ed. Weinheim: Wiley-VCH Verlag GmbH and Co. KGaA; 2006. ISBN: 3-527-31307-9

[4] Stein V, Nicoll RA. GABA generates excitement. Neuron. 2003;**37**:375-378

[5] Jonas P, Monyer H, editors. Handbook Ionotrophic Glutamate receptors in the CNS. Berlin, Hedelberg: Springer; 1999

[6] Jansen M, Dannhardt G. Antagonists and agonists at the glycine site of the NMDA receptors for therapeutic interventions. European Journal of Medicinal Chemistry. 2003;**38**:661-670

[7] Nicoll RA. Expression mechanisms underlying long-term potentiation: A postsynaptic view. Philosophical Transactions of the Royal Society, B: Biological Sciences. 2003;**358**:721-726

[8] Bazemore A, Elliott KA. Florey e factor i and gamma-aminobutyric acid. Nature. 1956;**178**:1052-1053

[9] Vannier C, Triller A. Biology of the postsynaptic receptor. International Review of Cytology. 1997;**176**:201-244

[10] Rajendra S, Lynch JW, Schofield PR. The glycine receptor. Pharmacology & Therapeutics. 1997;**73**:121-146

[11] Aprison MH, Daly EC. Biochemical aspects of transmission at inhibitory synapses: The role of glycine. Advances in Neurochemistry. 1978;**3**:203-294

[12] Li B et al. Differential regulation of synaptic and extrasynaptic NMDARs. Nature Neuroscience. 2002;**5**:833

[13] Kohr G. NMDAR function: Subunit composition versus spatial distribution. Cell and Tissue Research. 2006;**326**:439

Chapter 3

Trends of Protein Aggregation in Neurodegenerative Diseases

Abdulbaki Agbas

Abstract

Protein aggregation trends in neurodegenerative diseases are largely unmapped due to the complex nature of protein-protein interactions and their regulatory machineries such as protein proteolytic systems. Since the protein aggregation process in humans is a slow process, early determination of the patients that will develop neurodegenerative diseases later in life is critical in terms of starting effective treatment, which will reduce the expensive health care. In this chapter, I will discuss the nature of protein aggregation of signature proteins and the status of protein proteolytic systems such as proteasome and autophagosome in Alzheimer's disease, Parkinson's disease, amyotrophic lateral sclerosis, frontotemporal lobar degeneration, Huntington's disease, and prion disease under the light of recent studies including our new findings.

Keywords: protein aggregation, protein misfolding, neurodegenerative disease, aging, proteinopathy, amyloid plaque

1. Introduction

Extracellular deposits of protein aggregates are often relevant to human diseases in general. Protein aggregates are the product of misfolded proteins that escape from protein quality checkpoints such as the chaperon/chaperonin system, heat shock proteins (Hs90, Hs70, etc.), proteasomes, and the autophagosome system. They are mostly insoluble and tend to form amyloid plaques over time. In this chapter, I will review trends of protein aggregation in the most studied neurodegenerative diseases such as Alzheimer's disease (AD), amyotrophic lateral sclerosis (ALS), Parkinson's disease (PD), frontotemporal lobar degeneration (FTLD), prion, Huntington's disease, etc.

1.1 An overview for protein-folding

Biological self-assembly of proteins in a compact three-dimensional (3D) structure is the universal example of how the functional proteins can be separated from other biomolecules. This feature provides a functional advantage for proteins. 3D folding brings functional groups to close proximity creating a space where chemical reactions can occur; hence, the protein molecule becomes functional. Properly folded proteins need to maintain their stability which requires naturally interacting partners during their life term [1]. Failure of this native environment-protein interaction can lead to a wide variety of pathological conditions called *proteinopathy.*

Approximately 30 or more structurally different proteins have the potential to form an amyloid structure. Although there is no obvious homology in their primary structure, they all share a beta-pleated sheet (β-structure) as a polymer scaffold [3].

1.2 Energy landscape in protein-folding

Proteins in their native state, under the physiological conditions, are in a low energy state which provides thermodynamic stability [4]. With a large number of permutations, a systematic search for a stable polypeptide chain requires an enormous length of time ($\sim 1.6 \times 10^{15}$ trillion years). This makes it clear that the protein-folding process does not involve sequential steps. Cyrus Levinthal's calculation known as *Levinthal's paradox* reveals that proteins do not follow a folding process by trying every possible conformation; instead, they follow a partially defined pathway consisting of intermediates between fully denatured protein and its native structure (**Figure 1**) [1]. Two basic questions have not yet been answered: (i) what determines the correct folding state from the intermediate stage and (ii) how is the energy landscape unique to a specific protein-folding? Folding characteristics of small proteins (~100 amino acid residue) provide invaluable information about the amino acid sequence and energy landscape. A specific mutation in an amino acid sequence may provide critical information about the folding and unfolding kinetics [5]. Therefore, the energy landscape of certain signature proteins in neurodegenerative diseases may provide some critical information about the trends of such proteins that misfold and form aggregate. The problem lies on how to study the specific energy landscape of such proteins that are obtained from the patients (AD, ALS, PD, Creutzfeldt-Jakob disease, and Huntington's disease), which will predict the aggregate formation of the proteins. This will help in designing new drugs that either postpone or eliminate such aggregate formations; consequently, treatment options for neurodegenerative diseases may be possible.

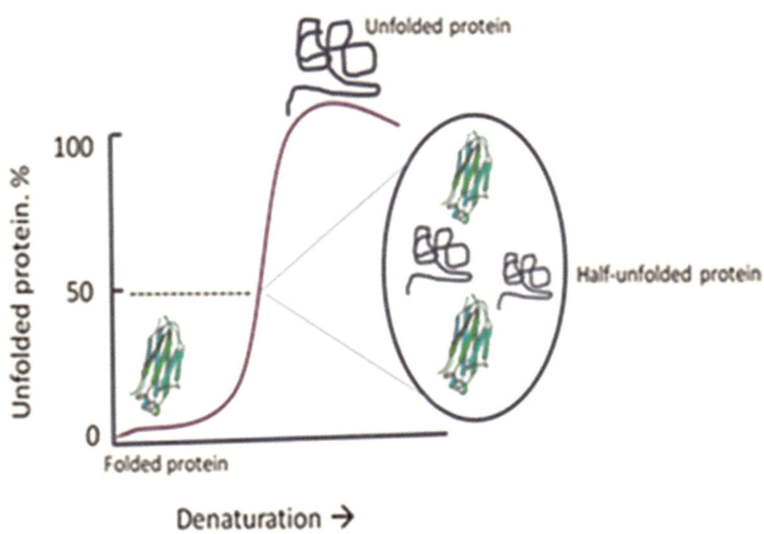

Figure 1.
Components of a partially denatured protein solution. In a half-unfolded protein solution, half of the protein species are fully folded and the other half are unfolded. This is an experimental condition; therefore, it is not known whether same or similar condition is existing in biology. The image is redrawn from 6th Edition of Biochemistry [1].

1.3 Protein misfolding in the cell

Although protein-folding principles are universal, the protein-folding environment needs to be taken into consideration in order to comprehend the protein-misfolding event. Some protein-folding is co-translational; they are initiated before leaving the ribosomal machinery upon completion of primary structure [6]. Most proteins undergo proper folding process in the cytoplasm after they leave the ribosome "quality control checkpoints" and began to interact with chaperones and heat shock proteins (HSPs). Recent studies reveal that molecular chaperones are essential not only in preventing misfolding but also in rescuing misfolded proteins even in their early stage of aggregation enabling them to have a "second chance" to fold correctly; this process requires ATP [7, 8]. Increased concentration of chaperone molecules and HSPs during cellular stress supports the notion that ATP is required [9]. Chaperonins, a subclass of chaperones, are the preferred molecules participating in the protein-folding process [10–12]. A possible chaperonin-naïve protein adverse interaction may very well initiate protein misfolding that will lead to protein aggregation. There are other proteins that complete their folding process in certain organelles such as the endoplasmic reticulum (ER) and mitochondria after being translocated into these organelles [7, 8]. The ER contains a large repertoire of molecular chaperons and folding catalysts [13, 14], making this organelle a major folding site and also the source of misfolded protein-related diseases [15]. Such organelles may utilize internal signals that allow certain proteins to penetrate into cell organelles to complete their folding. Wang et al. [16] recently demonstrated that a nuclear protein transactive response DNA-binding protein 43 kDa (TDP-43) penetrates into mitochondria using such internal signals and binds, preferably mitochondria-transcribed mRNA that encodes respiratory complex-I subunits (ND3 and ND6). This subsequently interferes with the proper assembly of complex-I and mitochondrial functions causing them to be impaired. The mitochondrial Hsp60/Hsp10 chaperonin system is essential for proper folding of proteins that are transported from cytosol to the inside of mitochondria via porins, and any mutation on this mitochondrial chaperonin system could be associated with neurodegenerative diseases [17].

Many misfolded proteins that escaped the "quality control checkpoints" have exposed regions that are normally buried in the hydrophobic core of the protein. Such regions could inappropriately interact with other macromolecules within the crowded bioenvironment of the cytosol [18]. This leads to the initiation of protein aggregation that may be the foundation of protein-relevant disease, proteinopathy. The readers should have a broad perspective of diverse process like translocation across the membranes, trafficking, secretion, the immune response, and regulation of the cell cycle that are dependent on the protein-folding mechanism [19]. Any failure of proper folding or the escape from quality control checkpoints gives rise to cell malfunctioning and, hence, to development of a proteinopathy [20, 21]. Protein propensity can determine the probability of misfolded protein that has a relatively higher extracellular milieu. Such protein propensity can be analyzed by employing **P**redictors **o**f **N**aturally **D**isordered **R**egions (PONDR) analysis. A few representatives of neurodegenerative disease hallmark proteins' PONDR® analysis were performed based on their primary amino acid sequence, and the results were shown in **Figure 2**. All four proteins possess reasonably high levels of disorder region that makes the protein a good candidate to undergo aggregation process once the necessary environmental conditions are achieved.

Protein misfolding is likely to initiate the formation of the seed for aggregation. Therefore, researchers have studied the protein-folding chaperone machinery and HSPs in the context of neurodegenerative disease [22]. Mutant Cu/Zn superoxide

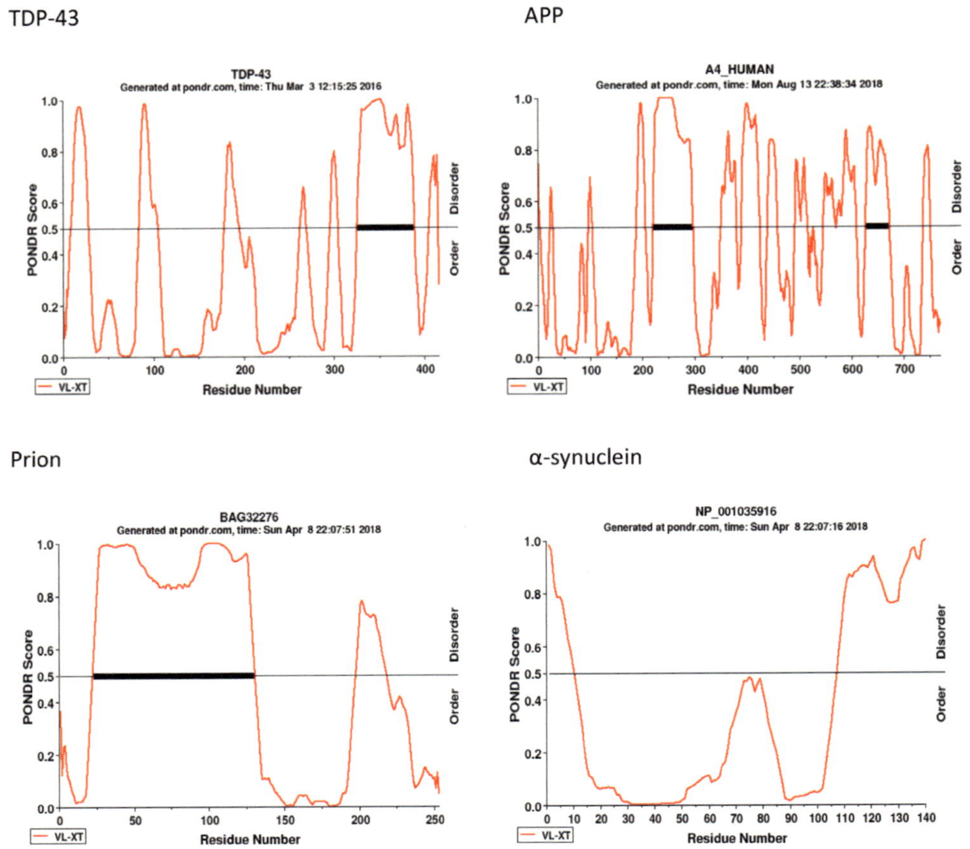

Figure 2.
Prediction analysis of some of the signature proteins for neurodegenerative diseases. PONDR® score predicts the disorder probability for a given protein or polypeptide based on the amino acid sequence. Disordered regions are defined as the entire proteins or regions of proteins that lack a fixed tertiary structure. These figures represent disordered regions of major proteins in neurodegenerative diseases. The black rectangle on the 0.5 line indicates the region that was visible in the crystal structure with this protein bound to its binding partner (www.molecularkinetics.com; main@molecularkinetics.com) under license from the WSU Research Foundation. PONDR® is copyright C_1999 by the WSU Research Foundation, all rights reserved*)*.

dismutase ($SOD1^{G93A}$) abundant in motor neurons and HSP interactions was studied. The proposal was made and experimentally demonstrated that mutant SOD1 binding to HSPs (Hsp70 and Hsp25) makes this chaperone unavailable for their anti-apoptotic functions and eventually leads to motor neuron death [23]. Our laboratory has also demonstrated both in vitro and in vivo that mutant SOD1 failed to bind calcineurin (CaN) in a fashion that CaN lost its activity [24]. This failed interaction may yield the accumulation of hyper-phosphorylated protein aggregations [25] since CaN is one of the Ser-/Thr-specific phosphatase that removes the phosphate from proteins [26]. Under the light of existing literature, it is now known that a number of diseases such as AD, PD, prion disease, and typ. 2 diabetes are directly relevant to aberrant proteins that escaped from chaperone quality check system and form insoluble aggregates [21, 27–29].

1.3.1 Amyloid formation

Filament-like (fibrous) protein aggregates are generally referred to as amyloid. The word *amyloid* indicates a starch-like compound. It is an accepted term for a group of conformational disorders. About 30 or so proteins have the tendency to form amyloid structure, and they are involved in the well-defined amyloidosis

(*amyloidosis*: abnormal proteins called amyloids buildup in the tissue). Although there is no consensus homology in their amino acid sequence and molecular details of amyloid fibrils have some commonalities, among them are as follows: (i) all share β-sheet as a polymer scaffold; (ii) all show specific optical behavior on binding dye molecule Congo red, displaying long-unbranched and often twisted structures; and (iii) a characteristic cross-beta X-ray fiber differentiation pattern [3, 30]. Sequence characteristics of certain regions, especially at either N- or C-terminal, may predict the protein propensity to form amyloid fibrils. PONDR® (**Figure 2**) analysis shows known neurodegenerative disease protein's tendency to form amyloid fibers. The idea that the relative aggregate rates for a wide range of polypeptides and proteins correlate with the physicochemical features of the molecules such as charge, secondary structure propensities, and hydrophobicity [31] was experimentally supported.

It is now known that polypeptides or proteins that have propensity for β-pleated structure have a tendency to form amyloid plaques. These β-pleated-enriched proteins fall to the lowest energy level in the energy landscape (**Figure 3**), and they are more hydrophobic. Consider a globular protein; the main polypeptide chain and hydrophobic regions are buried in the core of the protein. When these regions are exposed to more hydrophilic environment due to partial unfolding caused by low pH, proteolytic fragmentation, etc., conversion to amyloid fibrillation becomes possible [9]. Amyloid fibril formation takes years before it reveals clinical manifestation, and the fibril formation follows a lag phase followed by a period of rapid growth [32, 33]. The fibril structure is measurable and determinable by laboratory techniques; however, it requires postmortem tissues. It is now critical to develop some approaches that utilize less invasively obtained biosamples (e.g., blood) so that protein fibrillation may be monitored and fibril formation can be restrained with at early stages as part of early treatment option.

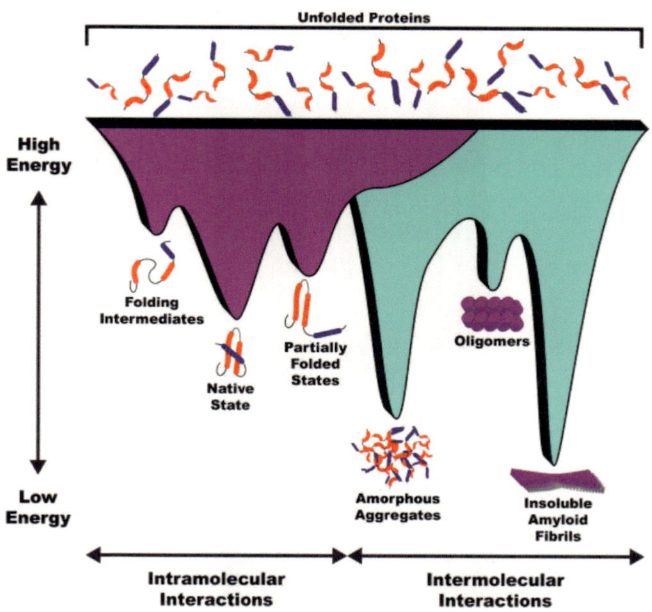

Figure 3.
Energy landscape of protein folding and aggregation. The purple surface shows possibility of the conformations leading to the thermodynamically balanced state (native state). Cyan-colored area of the landscape indicates the conformations moving toward to amorphous aggregates of insoluble amyloid fibrils (adopted and redrawn, Vabulas et al. [34].

1.3.2 Proteolysis-generated toxic protein species

Thermodynamic stability of a protein and its conformational kinetic determines the state of proper folding. Amyloid fibrils maintain the thermodynamically stable conformation in a highly organized hydrogen-bonded structure that is insoluble in aqueous media. This structure takes many years to progressively build up in tissues. Cellular homeostasis recognizes this event as toxic event and begins to encapsulate the amyloid fibrils in a plaque formation as part of the cellular defense mechanism. This plaque formation slows down and can eliminate further growth of the subsequent conversion of additional quantities of the same protein into amyloid fibrils [9]. However, readers should be aware that there are some naturally occurring nonpathogenic amyloid-like fibril formations such as the nanostructure of certain bacteria [35] and the mammalian melanocyte integral membrane protein [36]. The pathogenesis of amyloidogenic proteinopathy may be initiated with amyloidogenic peptide fragments by one or more proteases [37]. Human amyloid pathologies known to require proteolytic processing of a precursor protein include AD where Aβ peptide fragments are liberated from a large APP precursor protein by β- and γ-secretases [38]. A new potential biomarker for AD TDP-43 [39] may be involved in activating β-secretase that will generate Aβ peptide fragments [2]. **Figure 4** illustrates a simplified diagram of APP processing [2]. Modulation of Aβ generation by bio-metals was studied in both cell-free and cell-based assays. It was found that zinc (Zn^{2+}) ion induces APP-C99 dimerization, which prevents APP cleavage by γ-secretase and Aβ production [40]. The same group reported that copper (Cu^{2+}) ion was a γ-secretase inhibitor affecting APP processing [40]. These findings may suggest that the metal dyshomeostasis is a critical issue in generation of toxic protein species.

1.3.3 Proteasome malfunctioning

The β-sheet structure-enriched amyloid fibril formation relevant to protein aggregation is tightly controlled by molecular chaperones and the proteasome machinery. The proteasome is a large multisubunit complex that can be analogous to a food waste disposer. The proper function of such system is absolutely necessary for maintaining cell homeostasis [41].

It is expected that any proteasomal abnormalities may contribute to misfolding and protein aggregation diseases [42, 43]. In a pilot study, we observed that proteasome activity levels were reduced in plasma/platelet obtained from AD and ALS patients (**Figure 5**), while TDP-43 protein levels were increased in platelets

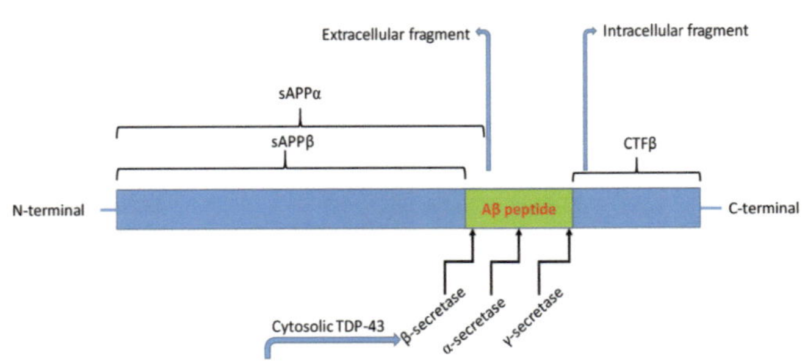

Figure 4.
Simplified diagram of APP structure and processing. APP undergoes sequential proteolysis by β-secretase, α-secretase, and γ-secretase for the release of Aβ from the neuronal plasma membrane. TDP-43 has been shown to increase intraneuronal Aβ accumulation via increased β-secretase activation (adapted and modified from Ref. [2]).

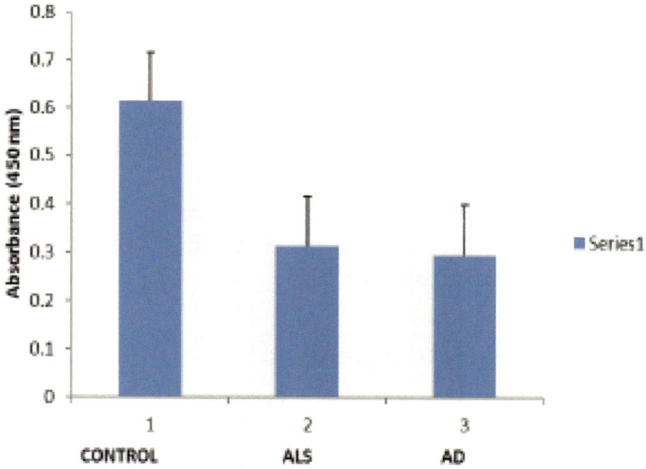

Figure 5.
Proteasome activity measurements in plasma. Extracellular proteasome activity levels were measured by proteasome 20S assay fluorogenic system (Enzo Biochem Inc. cat#BML-AK740-0001) designed to measure chymotrypsin-like protease activity of purified 20S proteasome. The detection of proteolytic activity is based on the release of three fluorogenic peptides. About 50% decrease in proteasome activity were observed in AD and ALS patient plasma (n = 3) (unpublished data).

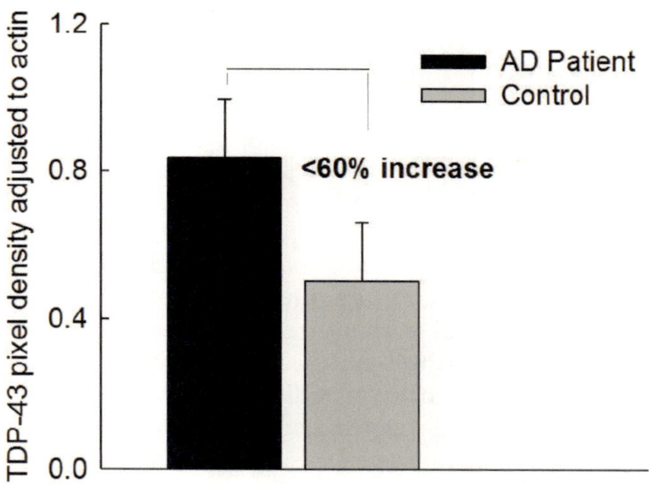

Figure 6.
Platelet lysate TDP-43 profile. TDP-43 protein levels were determined in platelet lysate by Western blotting method with a TDP-43 Ab (1:1000 dilution). Blood samples were obtained from AD patients (n = 3) and age-matched healthy subject (n = 3). Approximately <60% increase were observed in TDP-43 levels in AD patients (the figure was reproduced by permission [39]).

obtained from AD patients (**Figure 6**). This suggests that proteasome machinery was either malfunctioning or overwhelmed due to massive protein aggregation. Proteasome activity measurements in human plasma were successfully performed as a useful potential marker for various malignant and nonmalignant diseases [44]. Amyloid fibril formation that leads to abnormal protein aggregation may result in two functional consequences: (i) a toxic gain of function and (ii) a loss of function of the protein in question. Although the mature and organized protein fibrils are usually benign [32, 45], it is not well documented how disordered amyloid fibrils are being converted to malfunctioned protein species. One thought would be that the nonnative hydrophobic surfaces of the aberrant protein's interaction with cell membrane or other cellular components may initiate cell death [46].

2. Trends for misfolded proteins lead to neurodegeneration

Insoluble extracellular protein deposits in various human diseases have been recognized for a long time. Many proteins that have a tendency to be misfolded do form aggregates that initiate cellular dysfunction [47]. This section discusses how the proteins involved in neurodegenerative disease have a tendency to misfold. If we comprehend the biochemical and biophysical behavior of the proteins and their misfolding features, we will have a better understanding of proteinopathy and relevance to neurodegenerative diseases.

2.1 Common protein behavior in aggregation

In the last 25 years or so, many diseases have been linked to protein-misfolding cases, although their etiology of such diseases is different. In this section, the focus will be on neurodegenerative diseases because of the following reasons: (i) they are progressive, (ii) early diagnosis for these diseases are not available yet, (iii) they are not effectively treatable, and (iv) they inflict enormous personal, societal, and economic burdens. Some of them are aging relevant such as AD and PD; some of them are not like ALS, Creutzfeldt-Jakob disease (mad cow disease), and other human prion diseases (e.g., variant Creutzfeldt-Jakob diseases, Gerstmann-Straussler-Scheinker syndrome, fatal familial insomnia, and kuru).

Specific polypeptides that go into aggregation are different in each amyloidosis; however, there is a common feature in the behavior of these proteins; they all present enriched β-sheet structure. Such proteins are normally soluble in cytosol and in extracellular environment; however, somehow they progress into β-sheet-enriched insoluble filamentous polymers [47]. Not all β-structure-enriched insoluble filaments are an amyloid in nature. For example, some forms of SOD1-ALS are a conformational disease which involves amorphous aggregation of misfolded SOD1 [16, 48]. That is to say, the common structural motif in all amyloid fibers consists of cross-β-sheets. It is not uncommon that normally soluble proteins can undergo β-sheet-enriched conformational rearrangement and they tend to be more insoluble in nature. The concept of the β-sheet-enriched protein aggregation now becomes a common trend for polypeptide chains regardless of amino acid sequence [27]. The causes for the initiation of protein aggregation are not well documented; however, oxidative stress-induced reactive oxygen species (ROS) may be involved due to the role of ROS in several pathological disorders and aging [49, 50]. For example, glycine (Gly) residues are particularly susceptible for loss of a hydrogen ion, which results in the formation of Gly radical on the protein backbone which destabilizes protein structure [51]. Consequently, buried hydrophobic regions of the protein are exposed to the aqueous environment, and β-sheet structure formation is enhanced. These newly formed β-sheet structures link with that of neighboring structure which leads to the formation of a "seed" that eventually produces an aggregate [1].

2.2 Milestones for aggregate formation

Another characteristic in protein-folding disorders is a prolonged period in aggregate/plaque formation before clinical manifestation becomes obvious [47]. In aging-dependent neurodegenerative diseases such as AD and PD, aggregate/plaque formation is a lengthy process, while in ALS, SOD1, and TDP-43, aggregates are formed in the middle [52] or even younger ages [53]. One explanation for a lengthy process would be that the initial nucleation of a misfolded protein is very small and energetically stays in the upper level of the energy landscape (see **Figure 3**).

Therefore, the growth of the protein aggregate seed is kinetically unfavorable; hence, recruitment of new aberrant proteins for aggregate formation takes a longer period of time [54, 55]. Once the nucleation achieves a critical mass, the fibril formation and subsequent plaque formation become accelerated. This is why clinical manifestation of amyloidoses relevant to neurodegenerative disease mostly appears in old age. This is mostly true for sporadic AD; however, in familial AD, which represents only 5–10% of the total AD population, the disease onset tends to occur at the middle age (50 and above). In Down syndrome, β-amyloid precursor protein (APP), is encoded on chromosome 21 [47]. Patients with trisomy 21 develop abundant Aβ aggregates in the brain at younger age. Therefore, the lifelong aggregate formation is inevitable in Down syndrome patients, which supports the notion that Down syndrome patients are at high risk in developing AD. In the USA, it is estimated that more than a quarter million individuals live with Down syndrome and all will develop AD pathology as early as in their 30s [56]. In summary, protein aggregate formation starts at an early stage of life. This process is quicker in individuals with genetic conditions. Others display clinical signs at an old age as part of aging process.

2.3 Regional protein aggregation

Cellular misfolded proteins are inclined to accumulate in nearby organs, in a preferred cell type in a particular tissue [57], and in a particular cell organelle [58]. Although these proteins are distributed in systemic circulation, high concentrations can be maintained in organs. For example, Aβ fragments deposition in brain regions of AD patient, SOD1 and TDP-43 accumulation in spinal cord of ALS patients, and α-synuclein plaques in brain regions (neocortex, hippocampus, substantia nigra, thalamus, and cerebellum) of PD patients. Appearance of signature proteins (i.e., SOD1, TDP-43, α-synuclein, Aβ fragments, etc.) in systemic circulation supports the development of a surrogate biomarker in the blood when tissue sampling is not accessible [39].

It is interesting to note that misfolded aberrant proteins interact with apoptotic proteins in organ-specific organelle. Pasinelli et al. have demonstrated that anti-apoptotic protein Bcl-2 binds to detergent-insoluble mutant SOD1 ($SOD1^{G93A}$) protein aggregates that are present in mitochondria from the spinal cord but not in the liver in both mice and humans [58]. This observation suggests that misfolded aberrant protein functions are location specific. Valentine has reviewed studies on mutant SOD1 fragmentation in the Golgi apparatus, which may reveal early molecular signals before the onset of ALS symptoms [59]. There are more emerging studies in which emphasizing the region-specific protein aggregation can be considered a discriminatory signature in neurodegenerative diseases [60].

2.4 Systemic amyloidosis

The circulating proteins that have the potential to form extracellular amyloid deposits in multiple organs have been recently reviewed [47]. Local production of amyloid and non-amyloid protein species achieves the critical concentration for oligomerization and fibrillogenesis in specific organs. For example, Aβ deposition appears specifically in the brain tissue in AD. The Cu/Zn superoxide dismutase (SOD1) and TDP-43 deposition are measurable in brain and spinal cord tissues in ALS. These signature proteins can also be measurable in systemic circulation (**Table 1**).

We have recently published a paper describing platelet TDP-43 measurements as a proxy for brain tissue TDP-43 levels in AD patients [39]. This approach will aid

Clinical syndrome	Fibril species
Alzheimer's disease	Aβ fragments ($A\beta_{36\text{-}43}$) in brain
Spongiform encephalopathies (mad cow disease)	Prion protein fragments in brain
ALS	Spinal cord and brain region (movement control region,)
Hereditary cerebral hemorrhage with amyloidosis	Amyloid β –peptide or cystatin C
Huntington disease	HTTExon1
Parkinson's disease	α-synuclein

Table 1.
Extracellular fibril types in disease

to monitor the progress of aberrant protein aggregation in neurodegenerative diseases.

In age-related neurodegenerative diseases, it is quite common to observe β-sheet-enriched protein aggregates that are mostly detergent-insoluble. These insoluble protein aggregates tend to accumulate inside the cell; however, ultra-structure analysis of these aggregates may not be the same as that of extracellular amyloid fibrils. The commonality of these aggregate-forming proteins was discussed earlier (Section 1.3.1). Therefore, it is reasonably acceptable to classify the aberrant protein aggregation-related neurodegenerative diseases as a special form of amyloidosis [47].

Protein misfolding and subsequent aggregation are central in neurodegenerative diseases; however, the protein behavior in forming aggregates is somehow disease specific. In case of the α-synuclein, this protein is natively folded and normally water soluble in the cell. In normal health conditions, α-synuclein participates in the maintenance of synaptic vesicle supplies at the presynaptic terminals [61]. In PD, this protein misfolds and accumulates in spherical filamentous structures called Lewy bodies. This encapsulated structure forms particularly in dopaminergic and noradrenergic brainstem neurons and causes premature cell death [62, 63]. Therefore, Lewy bodies become a signature pattern for PD. Polyglutamine repeat of corresponding proteins that are produced as the result of different mutant genes becomes a distinct pattern in Huntington's disease and several forms of familial spinocerebellar ataxia [64]. AD is the only brain disorder that displays the accumulation of amyloid forming proteins both extracellularly (Aβ fragments) and intracellularly (hyper-phosphorylated tau) [47]. The question would be whether hyper-phosphorylated tau neurofibrillary tangles or Aβ accumulation initiate AD. The amyloid cascade hypothesis has been the most studied model of molecular pathogenesis in AD. This is a long-debated issue in the scientific community which has polarized into two schools of thought: "Baptists" that believe Aβ accumulation is the starting event or "Tauist" that believes that tau-relevant neurofibrillary tangles are the initiators for AD [65]. However, inherited mutations in tau protein do not directly lead to AD; yet, it causes another devastating disorder, FTLD with PD [66]. It is now more probable that inherited mutations in APP or in one of the APP cleaving proteases (e.g., presenilin/γ-secretase) cause aggressive early onset forms of AD [67].

What are the initiation factors in sporadic AD which makes about 5–10% of all AD cases? Not much is known so far. A new player in AD field is TDP-43 protein which induces intramural Aβ accumulation via increasing β-secretase (BACE-1) [2]. As it can be seen in **Figure 4**, TDP-43 acts on an upstream in the APP structure and may induce β-secretase. A ripple effect may induce to generate toxic Aβ fragments.

Levels of γ- and β-secretase activities are greater in brain tissue samples from AD patients than non-demented control subjects [68, 69]. Experimental studies conducted on 3xTg-AD (swAPP, PS1-M146V, tau-P301L) demonstrate that BACE-1 activity levels were elevated in the brain tissue and γ-secretase inhibitors reduced the BACE-1 activity, suggesting that γ-secretase mediates oxidative stress-induced expression of BACE-1 resulting in excessive Aβ production in AD [70]. Extracellular cleavage of APP by BACE-1 creates a soluble extracellular fragment and a cell membrane-bound fragment referred to as C99. Cleavage of C99 within its transmembrane domain by γ-secretase releases the intracellular domain of APP and produces Aβ. Since γ-secretase cleaves APP closer to the cell membrane than BACE1 does, it removes a fragment of the Aβ peptide. Initial cleavage of APP by α-secretase rather than BACE-1 prevents eventual generation of Aβ [71]. It is clear that the most notable neurodegenerative diseases (i.e., AD, ALS, FTLD, and PD) share a common prominent pathological feature, TDP-43 proteinopathy. This issue has been recently reviewed, and possibility of targeting TDP-43 as a common therapeutic approach to formulate a treatment for neurodegenerative diseases was discussed [72]. In our laboratory, we are also working on an assay methodology that uses peripheral blood-derived platelet TDP-43 profile that may help for early diagnosis of such diseases so that early treatment options could be available [39].

2.5 Aging and protein aggregation

Aging is the normal biological process that includes increased protein misfolding and aggregation process due to either reduced levels of quality control checkpoints such as chaperone system or proteasome complex. The proteins that form orderly (amyloid fibers) and disorderly (amorphous aggregates and plaques) show some common and essential biochemical and biophysical features that were discussed earlier. Therefore, such age-related neurodegenerative diseases may be considered a special form of amyloidoses [47]. The biochemical processes in aging are contributing to free radical-induced protein oxidation; hence, unnatural disulfide bridge formations can contribute oxidized protein aggregation as well [73] . Dismutase metalloenzyme (e.g., SOD1 and SOD2) activity levels are also reduced in aging [74, 75]. This contributes the inefficient removal of reactive oxygen ions; hence, more protein oxidation events take place, and subsequently protein aggregation occurs. Principal unanswered questions about these neurodegenerative disorders remain: how preciously native soluble proteins undergo partial unfolding, and does aberrant refolding produce highly stable polypeptide polymers? We can still make some predictions about the propensity of a given protein through PONDR® analysis. This publicly available online prediction program (www.pondr.com) can be utilized for predicting which regions of the protein will be more susceptible for disorderliness which may increase the chance of aberrant protein refolding [76, 77]. It is clear that time and supraphysiological concentrations of predictable pro-aggregate proteins are two important parameters in aggregation process. Other factors such as oxidizable amino acids (e.g., cysteine and methionine), population, local pH, and higher hydrophobic propensity of the protein help the oligomerization process. Equilibrium between natively folded protein and aberrant-folded protein can last for a long period of time. One approach would be that molten globule-like intermediates have persistent structure in unstable α-structure. Stable β-structure of the protein provides a template (seed) for the recruitment of additional peptide chains through physical interaction of those two structural regions of the protein. Finally, new hydrogen bonds form and stabilize the protein in an insoluble amyloid fibril [78, 79]. On the other hand, fibril deposition is not a necessary feature in prion disease. NMR structure of a domain of prion protein (PrR(121–231)) indicates that mutated amino acids in prion protein are involved in the maintenance of the hydrophobic core [80]. Exactly, how prion conversion propagates? The disease is currently under study [46]. As mentioned in Section 1.3, the ER contains a large repertoire of molecular chaperones and folding catalysts [13, 14]. The ER protein-folding system is also affected by aging process, and less fold-assisting proteins would be available; hence, unfolded and misfolded protein levels would be expected to be high. Two of the unconventional ER chaperone molecules are calnexin (Cnx) and calreticulin (Crt) [81–83] as cited in [84]. In a pilot study, we demonstrated that Cnx levels were reduced in aging rat brain as well as in neuronal cell culture (**Figure** 7). This observation supports the other works published in literature stating that protein-folding mechanisms are less efficient; therefore, aberrant-misfolded proteins rise and form aggregates.

2.6 Misfolded aberrant proteins cause cell dysfunction

Dynamic equilibrium between misfolded and natively folded proteins may be shifted in favor of protein misfolding and oligomerization in proteinopathy. No definite amyloid fibrils are seen in diseases, suggesting that smaller diffusible toxic protein species consisting of dimers, trimers, tetramers, and large oligomers may be involved in cell cytotoxicity [47]. Therefore, forming a plaque or aggregate may be considered a defense mechanism of cell against recruitment of more toxic protein species. The aggregate in plaque no longer poses toxicity for cell life; however, having such foreign structure in the cytosol or in extracellular milieu brings some serious problems in cell homeostasis. For example, the plaques are insoluble and indestructible by ubiquitinated proteasome system. The increased population of such aggregates may overwhelm or even block the proteasome machinery. Therefore, proteasome either slows down or becomes less functional. We have observed such reduced proteasome activity in AD and ALS cases (**Figure** 5).

Another interference of such toxic protein species is that they nonspecifically bind to receptors and channel proteins on the plasma membrane, thus interfering with numerous cell-signaling events [16, 85]. Mitochondrion homeostasis should be

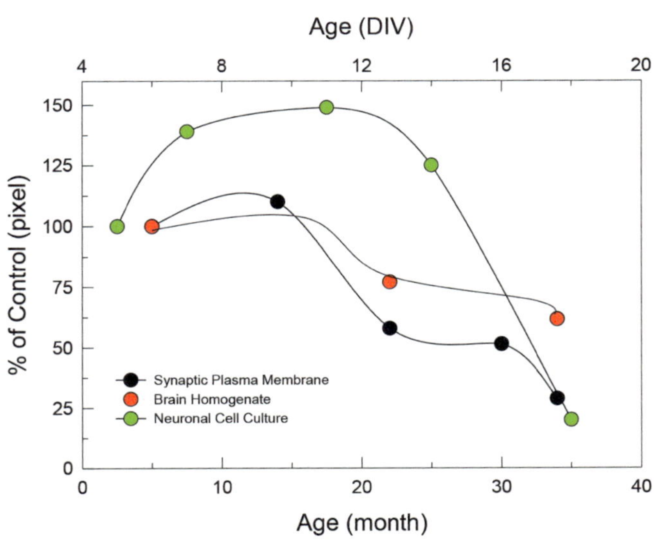

Figure 7.
Calnexin protein levels in aging. Calnexin protein levels were analyzed by Western blotting. Cnx levels were reduced during the aging process in total brain homogenate, synaptic plasma membrane, and neuronal cell culture. All samples were prepared from rat (n = 3) (unpublished data).

taken into consideration as well. Many mitochondrial proteins are nuclear-coded and transported into mitochondria [86]. These proteins are being transferred into mitochondria via outer membrane pores. Although these pores are specific, such small toxic protein species can nonspecifically bind the pores and slow down the protein entries into mitochondria if not completely block. Consequently, energy production mechanism of mitochondria may be compromised. Such hypothetical ideas need to be experimentally tested and should provide more convincing data about the cytotoxic effects of such protein species. Misfolded protein species get involved in apoptosis induction. Pasinelli et al. have reported that anti-apoptotic protein Bcl-2 interacts with both *wt* and mutant SOD1 ($SOD1^{G93A}$) [58]. This interaction induces apoptotic cascade because $SOD1^{G93A}$ mitochondria triggers apoptosis more strongly than the cytosolic mutant SOD1 [87].

3. Therapeutic approach to protein-misfolding disease

Proper protein-folding in the cell occurs either in the cytoplasm or within the secretory pathway. Dobson has reviewed this concept in detail [9].The readers are referred to this review to attain more in-depth understanding of the protein-folding relevant issues. The trend of misfolding protein increases when part of the polypeptide chain does not participate in a proper folding process. However, there are mechanisms that are available for aiding protein-folding. Chaperones are the molecules that collaborate with misfolded proteins to give a polypeptide chain several opportunities to fold. ATP-dependent chaperone molecules are critical for ensuring accuracy in proper folding [88]. The lumen of the ER also participates in protein-folding process by modifying the secretory proteins while they are still associated with the ER [89]. Any of these mechanistic failures contribute misfolded protein accumulation. Despite the attempt to rescue misfolded proteins that are destined to form insoluble aggregates, *proteasomes*, protein aggregate removal machinery, degrade such proteins from the cell so that cell homeostasis be maintained.

Several other protein misfolding-relevant diseases are caused by conformational modifications in extracellular milieu. Protein quality control-check systems of the cell (chaperones and heat shock protein family) cannot be linked to such misfolded protein population because such aggregation formation does not take place in cytosol. However, recent studies demonstrate the presence of extracellular proteasome machinery [92–94]. It is not clear yet whether these extracellular proteasomes are in the same categories in that of cytosolic since a recent report demonstrated that such extracellular proteasomes structurally differ from their cytosolic counterparts [94].

The major representatives of such disorders are the amyloidoses, in which protein aggregation in the extracellular space is associated with the presence of malfunctioned protein molecules [37, 90]. The chaperone-like small molecules may have the potential to be included in the treatment options for amyloidoses [91]. The more knowledge we attain on how chaperones and heat shock proteins interact with protein-folding process the better design for small molecules would be feasible.

Folding process of proteins is an environment-dependent physicochemical process. Some proteins have a folding issue where protein-folding takes place (i.e., lysosomal enzymes) while the others are efficiently folded in the ER but misfolded and misassembled at the destination (i.e., amyloidogenic proteins). This knowledge is helping industry-academia partnership for developing pharmacological intervention that reduces the mutant protein production, increases the rate of clearance of misfolded/mildly aggregated proteins, and increases the native stability of the proteins.

4. Conclusions

The majority of non-treatable neurodegenerative diseases are related to misfolding protein-induced aggregation and insoluble plaque formation. This process is very slow which makes early diagnosis of neurodegenerative diseases almost impossible at this time. However, some predictive studies may help to identify the proteins that have a tendency to form amyloid plaques. To know protein behavior in various physiological conditions and environmental factors will contribute to designing disease-specific drugs that interfere the aggregation formation in neurodegenerative diseases.

Acknowledgements

This work is partially supported by an intramural grant provided by the Office of Research and Sponsored Programs (ORSP) at Kansas City University of Medicine and Biosciences. Cultured neuronal cells were provided by Dr. Asma Zaidi. I would like to thank Dr. E. Dora Krizsan-Agbas for her constructive criticism and Tuba Agbas for proofreading the manuscript.

Conflict of interest

The author declares no conflict of interest.

Author details

Abdulbaki Agbas
Department of Basic Sciences, Kansas City University of Medicine and Biosciences, Kansas City, MO, USA

*Address all correspondence to: aagbas@kcumb.edu

References

[1] Berg JM, Tymoczko JL, Stryer L. Biochemistry. 6th ed. USA: W.H. Freeman and Company; 2007

[2] Youmans KL, Wolozin B. TDP-43: A new player on the AD field? Experimental Neurology. 2012;**237**(1): 90-95

[3] Sigurdsson E, Calero M, Gasset M. Amyloid proteins. In: Methods in Molecular Biology, Vol. 849. 2nd ed. Springer; 2012

[4] Dinner AR et al. Understanding protein-folding via free-energy surfaces from theory and experiment. Trends in Biochemical Sciences. 2000;**25**(7): 331-339

[5] Fersht AR et al. Reconstruction by site-directed mutagenesis of the transition state for the activation of tyrosine by the tyrosyl-tRNA synthetase: A mobile loop envelopes the transition state in an induced-fit mechanism. Biochemistry. 1988;**27**(5): 1581-1587

[6] Hardesty B, Kramer G. Folding of a nascent peptide on the ribosome. Progress in Nucleic Acid Research and Molecular Biology. 2001;**66**:41-66

[7] Bukau B, Horwich AL. The Hsp70 and Hsp60 chaperone machines. Cell. 1998;**92**(3):351-366

[8] Hartl FU, Hayer-Hartl M. Molecular chaperones in the cytosol: From nascent chain to folded protein. Science. 2002; **295**(5561):1852-1858

[9] Dobson CM. Protein folding and misfolding. Nature. 2003;**426**(6968): 884-890

[10] Weiss C et al. Dynamic complexes in the chaperonin-mediated protein-folding cycle. Frontiers in Molecular Biosciences. 2016;**3**:80

[11] Gruber R, Horovitz A. Allosteric mechanisms in chaperonin machines. Chemical Reviews. 2016;**116**(11): 6588-6606

[12] Hayer-Hartl M, Bracher A, Hartl FU. The GroEL-GroES chaperonin machine: A nano-cage for protein-folding. Trends in Biochemical Sciences. 2016;**41**(1):62-76

[13] Hammond C, Helenius A. Quality control in the secretory pathway. Current Opinion in Cell Biology. 1995; **7**(4):523-529

[14] Kaufman RJ et al. The unfolded protein response in nutrient sensing and differentiation. Nature Reviews. Molecular Cell Biology. 2002;**3**(6): 411-421

[15] Chambers JE, Marciniak SJ. Cellular mechanisms of endoplasmic reticulum stress signaling in health and disease. 2. Protein misfolding and ER stress. American Journal of Physiology. Cell Physiology. 2014;**307**(8):C657-C670

[16] Wang W et al. The inhibition of TDP-43 mitochondrial localization blocks its neuronal toxicity. Nature Medicine. 2016;**22**(8):869-878

[17] Bross P, Magnoni R, Bie AS. Molecular chaperone disorders: Defective Hsp60 in neurodegeneration. Current Topics in Medicinal Chemistry. 2012;**12**(22):2491-2503

[18] Ellis RJ. Macromolecular crowding: An important but neglected aspect of the intracellular environment. Current Opinion in Structural Biology. 2001; **11**(1):114-119

[19] Radford SE, Dobson CM. From computer simulations to human disease: Emerging themes in protein-folding. Cell. 1999;**97**(3):291-298

[20] Thomas PJ, Qu BH, Pedersen PL. Defective protein-folding as a basis of human disease. Trends in Biochemical Sciences. 1995;**20**(11):456-459

[21] Horwich A. Protein aggregation in disease: A role for folding intermediates forming specific multimeric interactions. The Journal of Clinical Investigation. 2002;**110**(9):1221-1232

[22] Boillee S, Vande Velde C, Cleveland DW. ALS: A disease of motor neurons and their nonneuronal neighbors. Neuron. 2006;**52**(1):39-59

[23] Okado-Matsumoto A, Fridovich I. Amyotrophic lateral sclerosis: A proposed mechanism. Proceedings of the National Academy of Sciences of the United States of America. 2002;**99**(13): 9010-9014

[24] Agbas A et al. Activation of brain calcineurin (Cn) by Cu-Zn superoxide dismutase (SOD1) depends on direct SOD1-Cn protein interactions occurring in vitro and in vivo. The Biochemical Journal. 2007;**405**(1):51-59

[25] Kim JM et al. Impaired Cu-Zn superoxide dismutase (SOD1) and calcineurin (Cn) interaction in ALS: A presumed consequence for TDP-43 and zinc aggregation in Tg SOD1(G93A) rodent spinal cord tissue. Neurochemical Research. 2018. https://doi.org/10.1007/s11064-017-2461-z

[26] Hemenway CS, Heitman J. Calcineurin. Structure, function, and inhibition. Cell Biochemistry and Biophysics. 1999;**30**(1):115-151

[27] Dobson CM. The structural basis of protein-folding and its links with human disease. Philosophical Transactions of the Royal Society of London. Series B, Biological Sciences. 2001;**356**(1406): 133-145

[28] Tan SY, Pepys MB. Amyloidosis. Histopathology. 1994;**25**(5):403-414

[29] Kelly JW. The alternative conformations of amyloidogenic proteins and their multi-step assembly pathways. Current Opinion in Structural Biology. 1998;**8**(1):101-106

[30] Sunde M, Blake C. The structure of amyloid fibrils by electron microscopy and X-ray diffraction. Advances in Protein Chemistry. 1997;**50**:123-159

[31] Chiti F et al. Rationalization of the effects of mutations on peptide and protein aggregation rates. Nature. 2003; **424**(6950):805-808

[32] Caughey B, Lansbury PT. Protofibrils, pores, fibrils, and neurodegeneration: Separating the responsible protein aggregates from the innocent bystanders. Annual Review of Neuroscience. 2003;**26**:267-298

[33] Bitan G et al. Amyloid beta-protein (Abeta) assembly: Abeta 40 and Abeta 42 oligomerize through distinct pathways. Proceedings of the National Academy of Sciences of the United States of America. 2003;**100**(1):330-335

[34] Vabulas RM, Raychaudhuri S, Hayer-Hartl M, Hartl FU. Cold Spring Harbor Perspectives in Biology. 2010;**2** (12):a004390. DOI: 10.1101/cshperspect. a004390. Review

[35] Kelly JW. Alternative conformations of amyloidogenic proteins govern their behavior. Current Opinion in Structural Biology. 1996;**6**(1):11-17

[36] Kelly JW, Balch WE. Amyloid as a natural product. The Journal of Cell Biology. 2003;**161**(3):461-462

[37] Wilhite R et al. Platelet phosphorylated TDP-43: An exploratory study for a peripheral surrogate biomarker development for Alzheimer's disease. Future Science OA. 2017;**3**(4): FSO238

[38] Gerber H et al. Zinc and copper differentially modulate amyloid

precursor protein processing by gamma-secretase and amyloid-beta peptide production. The Journal of Biological Chemistry. 2017;**292**(9):3751-3767

[39] Goldberg AL. Protein degradation and protection against misfolded or damaged proteins. Nature. 2003; **426**(6968):895-899

[40] Bence NF, Sampat RM, Kopito RR. Impairment of the ubiquitin-proteasome system by protein aggregation. Science. 2001;**292**(5521): 1552-1555

[41] Macario AJ, Conway de Macario E. Sick chaperones and ageing: A perspective. Ageing Research Reviews. 2002;**1**(2):295-311

[42] Gorodkiewicz E, Ostrowska H, Sankiewicz A. SPR imaging biosensor for the 20S proteasome: Sensor development and application to measurement of proteasomes in human blood plasma. Mikrochimica Acta. 2011; **175**(1–2):177-184

[43] Walsh DM et al. Naturally secreted oligomers of amyloid beta protein potently inhibit hippocampal long-term potentiation in vivo. Nature. 2002; **416**(6880):535-539

[44] Sherman MY, Goldberg AL. Cellular defenses against unfolded proteins: A cell biologist thinks about neurodegenerative diseases. Neuron. 2001;**29**(1):15-32

[45] Selkoe DJ. Folding proteins in fatal ways. Nature. 2003;**426**(6968):900-904

[46] Kerman A et al. Amyotrophic lateral sclerosis is a non-amyloid disease in which extensive misfolding of SOD1 is unique to the familial form. Acta Neuropathologica. 2010;**119**(3): 335-344

[47] Stadtman ER. Protein oxidation and aging. Free Radical Research. 2006; **40**(12):1250-1258

[48] Zuo L, Motherwell MS. The impact of reactive oxygen species and genetic mitochondrial mutations in Parkinson's disease. Gene. 2013;**532**(1):18-23

[49] Owen MC et al. Protein stability and unfolding following glycine radical formation. Molecules. 2017;**22**(4), 655:1-18. https://doi.org/10.3390/molecules22040655

[50] Wijesekera LC, Leigh PN. Amyotrophic lateral sclerosis. Orphanet Journal of Rare Diseases. 2009;**4**:3

[51] Longinetti E et al. Physical and cognitive fitness in young adulthood and risk of amyotrophic lateral sclerosis at an early age. European Journal of Neurology. 2017;**24**(1):137-142

[52] Jarrett JT, Lansbury, Jr. PT. Seeding one-dimensional crystallization of amyloid: A pathogenic mechanism in Alzheimer's disease and scrapie? Cell. 1993;**73**(6):1055-1058

[53] Perutz MF, Windle AH. Cause of neural death in neurodegenerative diseases attributable to expansion of glutamine repeats. Nature. 2001; **412**(6843):143-144

[54] Hartley D et al. Down syndrome and Alzheimer's disease: Common pathways, common goals. Alzheimer's & Dementia. 2015;**11**(6):700-709

[55] Durham HD et al. Aggregation of mutant Cu/Zn superoxide dismutase proteins in a culture model of ALS. Journal of Neuropathology and Experimental Neurology. 1997;**56**(5): 523-530

[56] Pasinelli P et al. Amyotrophic lateral sclerosis-associated SOD1 mutant proteins bind and aggregate with Bcl-2 in spinal cord mitochondria. Neuron. 2004;**43**(1):19-30

[57] Valentine JS. Do oxidatively modified proteins cause ALS? Free

Radical Biology & Medicine. 2002; **33**(10):1314-1320

[58] Hekmatimoghaddam S, Zare-Khormizi MR, Pourrajab F. Underlying mechanisms and chemical/biochemical therapeutic approaches to ameliorate protein misfolding neurodegenerative diseases. BioFactors. 2017;**43**(6):737-759

[59] Diao J et al. Native alpha-synuclein induces clustering of synaptic-vesicle mimics via binding to phospholipids and synaptobrevin-2/VAMP2. eLife. 2013;**2**: e00592

[60] Miller DB, O'Callaghan JP. Biomarkers of Parkinson's disease: Present and future. Metabolism. 2015; **64**(3 Supp. 1):S40-S46

[61] Sutachan JJ et al. Cellular and molecular mechanisms of antioxidants in Parkinson's disease. Nutritional Neuroscience. 2012;**15**(3):120-126

[62] Zoghbi HY, Orr HT. Glutamine repeats and neurodegeneration. Annual Review of Neuroscience. 2000;**23**: 217-247

[63] Mudher A, Lovestone S. Alzheimer's disease-do tauists and baptists finally shake hands? Trends in Neurosciences. 2002;**25**(1):22-26

[64] Hutton M. Missense and splice site mutations in tau associated with FTDP-17: Multiple pathogenic mechanisms. Neurology. 2001;**56**(11 Supp. 4):S21-S25

[65] Selkoe DJ, Podlisny MB. Deciphering the genetic basis of Alzheimer's disease. Annual Review of Genomics and Human Genetics. 2002;**3**:67-99

[66] Kim JY et al. Distinct amyloid precursor protein processing machineries of the olfactory system. Biochemical and Biophysical Research Communications. 2018;**495**(1):533-538

[67] Shen Y et al. Increased plasma beta-secretase 1 may predict conversion to Alzheimer's disease dementia in individuals with mild cognitive impairment. Biological Psychiatry. 2018; **83**(5):447-455

[68] Jo DG et al. Evidence that gamma-secretase mediates oxidative stress-induced beta-secretase expression in Alzheimer's disease. Neurobiology of Aging. 2010;**31**(6):917-925

[69] Jonsson T et al. A mutation in APP protects against Alzheimer's disease and age-related cognitive decline. Nature. 2012;**488**(7409):96-99

[70] Gao J et al. Pathomechanisms of TDP-43 in neurodegeneration. Journal of Neurochemistry. 2018 Feb 27. DOI: 10.1111/jnc.14327. [Epub ahead of print] Review. PMID: 29486049

[71] Yu NT et al. Disulfide bond formation in the eye lens. Proceedings of the National Academy of Sciences of the United States of America. 1985; **82**(23):7965-7968

[72] Ozsoy O et al. The effect of ingested sulfite on visual evoked potentials, lipid peroxidation, and antioxidant status of brain in normal and sulfite oxidase-deficient aged rats. Toxicology and Industrial Health. 2016;**32**(7):1197-1207

[73] Salminen LE et al. Vulnerability of white matter tracts and cognition to the SOD2 polymorphism: A preliminary study of antioxidant defense genes in brain aging. Behavioural Brain Research. 2017;**329**:111-119

[74] Dunker AK et al. Intrinsically disordered protein. Journal of Molecular Graphics & Modelling. 2001;**19**(1): 26-59

[75] Garner E et al. Predicting binding regions within disordered proteins. Genome Informatics. 1999;**10**:41-50

[76] Booth DR et al. Instability, unfolding and aggregation of human lysozyme variants underlying amyloid

fibrillogenesis. Nature. 1997;**385**(6619): 787-793

[77] Radford SE, Dobson CM. Insights into protein-folding using physical techniques: Studies of lysozyme and alpha-lactalbumin. Philosophical Transactions of the Royal Society of London. Series B, Biological Sciences. 1995;**348**(1323):17-25

[78] Riek R et al. NMR structure of the mouse prion protein domain PrP(121–231). Nature. 1996;**382**(6587):180-182

[79] Williams DB. The Merck Frosst Award Lecture 1994/La conference Merck Frosst 1994. Calnexin: A molecular chaperone with a taste for carbohydrate. Biochemistry and Cell Biology. 1995;**73**(3–4):123-132

[80] Bergeron JJ et al. Calnexin: A membrane-bound chaperone of the endoplasmic reticulum. Trends in Biochemical Sciences. 1994;**19**(3): 124-128

[81] Michalak M et al. Calreticulin. The Biochemical Journal. 1992;**285**(Pt 3): 681-692

[82] Parodi AJ. Protein glucosylation and its role in protein-folding. Annual Review of Biochemistry. 2000;**69**:69-93

[83] Rusmini P et al. The role of the protein quality control system in SBMA. Journal of Molecular Neuroscience. 2016;**58**(3):348-364

[84] Stojanovski D, Bohnert M, Pfanner N, van der Laan M. Mechanisms of protein sorting in mitochondria. In: Wallace DCaYRJ, editor. Mitochondria. Cold Spring Harbor, New York: Cold Spring Harbor Laboratory Press; 2014. pp. 65-82

[85] Takeuchi H et al. Mitochondrial localization of mutant superoxide dismutase 1 triggers caspase-dependent cell death in a cellular model of familial amyotrophic lateral sclerosis. The Journal of Biological Chemistry. 2002; **277**(52):50966-50972

[86] Cohen FE, Kelly JW. Therapeutic approaches to protein-misfolding diseases. Nature. 2003;**426**(6968): 905-909

[87] Garcia-Huerta P et al. ER chaperones in neurodegenerative disease: Folding and beyond. Brain Research. 2016;**1648**(Pt B):580-587

[88] Rochet JC, Lansbury, Jr. PT. Amyloid fibrillogenesis: Themes and variations. Current Opinion in Structural Biology. 2000;**10**(1):60-68

[89] Chiti F, Dobson CM. Protein misfolding, amyloid formation, and human disease: A summary of progress over the last decade. Annual Review of Biochemistry. 2017;**86**:27-68

[90] Kulichkova VA et al. Proteomic analysis of affinity-purified extracellular proteasomes reveals exclusively 20S complexes. Oncotarget. 2017;**8**(60): 102134-102149

[91] Dianzani C et al. Extracellular proteasome-osteopontin circuit regulates cell migration with implications in multiple sclerosis. Scientific Reports. 2017;**7**:43718

[92] Tsimokha AS et al. Extracellular proteasomes are deficient in 19S subunits as revealed by iTRAQ quantitative proteomics. Journal of Cellular Physiology. 2017;**232**(4): 842-851

[93] Chapman MR et al. Role of *Escherichia coli* curli operons in directing amyloid fiber formation. Science. 2002; **295**(5556):851-855

[94] Berson JF et al. Proprotein convertase cleavage liberates a fibrillogenic fragment of a resident glycoprotein to initiate melanosome biogenesis. The Journal of Cell Biology. 2003;**161**(3):521-533

Chapter 4

Targeting the NO/cGMP/CREB Phosphorylation Signaling Pathway in Alzheimer's Disease

Jole Fiorito, Shi-Xian Deng, Donald W. Landry and Ottavio Arancio

Abstract

Alzheimer's disease (AD) is a progressive neurodegenerative disease and the most common form of senile dementia. Recently, scientists have put significant effort into exploring the molecular mechanisms involved in the pathological processes leading to the disease. A vast number of studies have focused on understanding the nitric oxide (NO) signaling pathway, which culminates with the phosphorylation of the transcription factor cAMP-responsive element-binding protein (CREB) through the increase of the second messenger cyclic guanosine monophosphate (cGMP) and activation of cGMP-dependent protein kinase. This book chapter provides an overview of the progress being made in modulating the hippocampal synaptic transmissions, which are critical for learning and memory, by targeting the different components of the NO/cGMP/CREB phosphorylation signaling pathway. Furthermore, a description of recent research on this pathway through the use of phosphodiesterase inhibitors is emphasized.

Keywords: Alzheimer's disease, nitric oxide, cyclic guanosine monophosphate, cGMP-dependent protein kinase, phosphodiesterases, phosphodiesterase inhibitors, cAMP-regulatory element-binding protein

1. Introduction

Alzheimer's disease (AD) is a progressive neurodegenerative disorder that involves cognitive impairment, such as loss of memory and reasoning and decline in mental ability. The AD brain is characterized by cell death and intra- and extracellular accumulation of amyloid-beta (Aβ) and tau proteins that form senile plaques and neurofibrillary tangles, respectively. Nowadays, medical treatments available on the market comprise two classes of drugs, acetylcholinesterase (AchE) inhibitors (i.e. donepezil, galantamine, and rivastigmine) and *N*-methyl-D-aspartate (NMDA) receptor antagonist (i.e. memantine). Based on the AD cholinergic hypothesis, acetylcholine-containing neurons project diffusely to the cortex and modulate cognitive processing. Damage of these projections has been associated with learning and memory impairment. Thus, AchE inhibitors block the acetylcholine-degrading enzyme consequently raising the levels of the acetylcholine neurotransmitter in the brain [1]. Differently from AchE inhibitors, memantine antagonizes the NMDA receptors, modulating dysfunctions in the glutamatergic neurotransmission associated to AD. Even if glutamate NMDA receptors are essential for synaptic transmission [2], excessive stimulation of glutamatergic signaling results in excitotoxicity, a condition in which nerve cells are damaged leading to gradual loss of synaptic function and ultimate neuronal cell death. Thus, memantine reduces glutamate excitotoxicity effects [3]. Although these medications have been used for decades, they help with cognitive and behavioral symptoms but fail stopping or reversing the progression of the disease. Because of this limitation, the discovery of new therapeutic strategies for the treatment of AD has become a critical and shared goal to academia and industry.

Much progress has been made since Aβ and tau proteins were recognized as the major hallmarks of AD. With the aim of finding novel and more effective therapeutic targets, scientists have put enormous effort in understanding the molecular mechanisms causing the development and progression of the disease. Long-term potentiation (LTP) is the primary experimental model for investigating synaptic transmission and strength in the hippocampus [2]. Changes in synaptic strength, resulting from specific patterns of synaptic activity, define the biological process called synaptic plasticity, which is thought to contribute to learning and memory [4]. It is widely recognized that LTP at the CA3-CA1 synapse is triggered by postsynaptic NMDA receptors in response to high-frequency synaptic transmission. During the induction of LTP, the depolarization of the postsynaptic membrane, induced by tetanic stimulation, removes the Mg^{2+} block from the NMDA receptor channel that would otherwise occupy the lumen of the channel at resting membrane potential levels. At the same time, the neurotransmitter L-glutamate is released to activate NMDA receptors, upon which Ca^{2+} as well as Na^{+} ions enter the dendritic spine. Consequently, the elevation of intracellular Ca^{2+} triggers LTP. The implication of the NMDA receptors in the process of LTP has been proven by a variety of NMDA antagonists, such as MK-801 and 2-amino-5-phosphopentanoate that are able to prevent the induction of LTP [2, 5]. Likewise, Ca^{2+} chelators injected intracellularly block the induction of LTP as demonstrated by Lynch and coworkers [6]. Ca^{2+} triggers activation of second messenger cascades relevant to memory formation such as the NO cascade [7] on which we have focused in this chapter. LTP has been used as an electrophysiological model to investigate the correlation between memory impairment and synaptic strengthening in hippocampal slices of mice and to evaluate the effect of various compounds on synaptic transmission. Interestingly, $A\beta_{1-42}$ has been found to block LTP through the disruption of different molecular pathways, such as the kinases c-Jun N-terminal kinase, cyclin-dependent kinase 5, and p38 mitogen-activated protein kinase (MAPK) as well as the metabotropic glutamate receptor type 5 [8], the extracellular signal-regulated kinase (ERK)-MAPK cascade [9], the cyclic adenosine monophosphate (cAMP)/cAMP-dependent-protein kinase/cAMP-regulatory element-binding protein (CREB) pathway [10], and the NO/cyclic guanosine monophosphate (cGMP)/CREB pathway [11].

This chapter provides an overview of the NO/cGMP/CREB phosphorylation signaling pathway and its role in learning and memory mechanisms during aging and neurodegenerative diseases. Several studies have demonstrated the association between NO, cGMP and CREB phosphorylation and synaptic plasticity [11–13]. The overall pathway includes the gaseous molecule NO, which is synthesized by the enzyme nitric oxide synthase (NOS) from arginine and induces an increase in the levels of second messenger cGMP by activating the enzyme soluble guanylyl cyclase (sGC). cGMP, consequently, activates the cGMP-dependent protein kinases (PKGs), a family of enzymes that is involved as transduction mediators in a number of cellular signaling systems. Lastly, PKGs phosphorylate the transcription factor CREB at its serine 166 (Ser-166), leading to the transcription of genes relevant to learning and memory during LTP. Additionally, phosphodiesterase enzymes (PDEs) act on the pathway by hydrolyzing cGMP and therefore lowering the intracellular levels of the second messenger (**Figure 1**). CREB phosphorylation has been recognized as a crucial event during synaptic plasticity. Indeed, not only does the increase of phosphorylated CREB (pCREB) levels regulate the transcription of important neuronal genes, such as the gene for brain-derived neurotrophic factor (BDNF) [14] but also leads to the generation of new dendritic spines that represent morphological changes crucial in LTP in central neurons [15]. The fundamental role of the NO/cGMP/CREB signaling pathway in strengthening the synaptic transmissions has been explored by observing the effect of inhibiting the single components of the pathway on CREB phosphorylation [16–18]. On the contrary, the stimulation of this pathway has shown to restore the levels of pCREB and improve age-related learning and memory in *in vivo* tests [19, 20]. Importantly, in the presence of Aβ protein the NO/cGMP/CREB pathway is inhibited. In fact, findings have shown that the increase of pCREB during synaptic plasticity is blocked by Aβ in cultured cortical and hippocampal neurons [10, 21] as well as in mouse hippocampal slices [11]. Furthermore, to correlate the molecular mechanisms involved during LTP to the cognitive functions of learning and memory *in vivo*, the NO/cGMP/CREB cascade has been explored in a variety of animal models using different memory-related tasks [11, 19].

Due to the high relevance of the NO/cGMP/CREB pathway in aging and neurodegenerative disorders, a growing number of studies have focused on developing therapeutic strategies aimed at regulating this signaling pathway. The following sections summarize the single components of the pathway and their implication in neurodegenerative disorders, with particular emphasis on AD, as well as the therapeutic approaches advanced for targeting each of these pathway

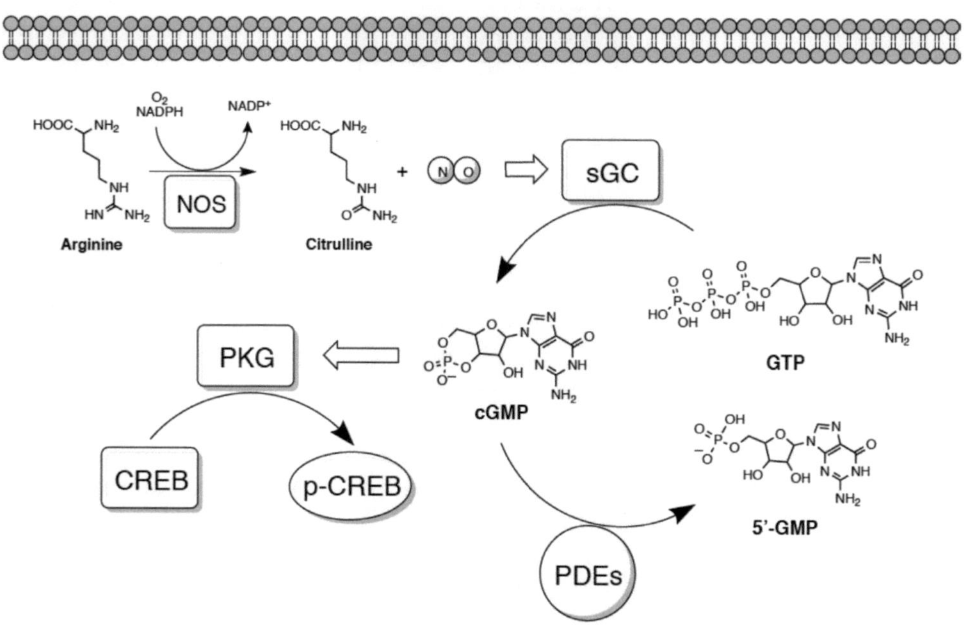

Figure 1.
NO/cGMP/CREB phosphorylation signaling pathway. Nitric oxide (NO) is produced during the conversion of arginine into citrulline by the enzyme nitric oxide synthase (NOS). NO activates soluble guanylyl cyclase (sGC), which stimulates cyclic guanosine monophosphate (cGMP) production from guanosine triphosphate (GTP). cGMP is degraded into 5'-GMP by the phosphodiesterases (PDEs). The increase of cGMP levels activates cGMP-dependent protein kinase (PKG), which induces phosphorylation of cAMP-responsive element binding (CREB).

effectors. Among them, inhibitors of PDEs have been the most studied and developed agents modulating the NO/cGMP/CREB pathway.

2. NO and NO donors

Nitric oxide, •N=O (abbreviated as NO) is a diatomic molecule with an unpaired electron in its outer orbit. NO is a highly diffusible gaseous molecule, which easily crosses cell membranes due to its high lipophilicity [22]. NO is involved in different metabolic pathways. NO can react with molecular oxygen (O_2) or superoxide anion ($O_2^{\bullet-}$) to produce nitrogen reactive species, including peroxynitrite [22–24]. At a cellular level, NO is a signaling molecule that regulates important processes such as cell differentiation and death, immune response, vascular tone and function, platelet aggregation, angiogenesis, and neurotransmission [25–27]. NO is predominantly produced along the biosynthetic process that converts the amino acid arginine into citrulline, in the presence of oxygen and cofactors (**Figure 1**). This metabolic pathway is catalyzed by nitric oxide synthases (NOS) [28, 29]. NOS occur in three isoforms: neuronal NOS (nNOS), endothelial NOS (eNOS), and inducible NOS (iNOS). nNOS and eNOS are constitutively expressed and their activities are regulated by calcium-bound calmodulin. Both constitutive NOS isoforms respond immediately to increased levels of calcium and produce low levels of NO rapidly. The endothelial isoform is a key regulator of NO production in vascular endothelial cells and has a major role in the regulation of vascular tone and platelet aggregation. In the brain, the basal concentration of NO is mainly regulated by nNOS and, in a smaller extent, by eNOS [28]. iNOS is tightly bound to calmodulin and acts independently of calcium levels; its activity is induced by a number of cytokines, such as interferon-gamma and tumor necrosis factor. While several studies have associated iNOS with the development of disease such as atherosclerosis, others have proposed that the activity of iNOS in pathological conditions has a protective mechanism [28, 30]. The main receptor for NO is sGC. The binding of NO to the heme Fe center present in the catalytic site increases the enzymatic basal activity for conversion of guanosine 5′-triphosphate (GTP) to cyclic guanosine monophosphate (cGMP) [31–33]. Most recently, Martin and coworkers have reported the mechanism of binding of NO to sGC [34]. By using isotopic ^{14}NO and ^{15}NO in rapid-freeze quench experiments, different intermediates of the complex NO–sGC were trapped and analyzed by electron paramagnetic resonance (EPR) spectroscopy. This study confirmed that NO binds to the distal side of heme Fe and then a second molecule of NO binds to the proximal side, leading to the release of NO from the distal side of the transient bis-NO-sGC complex. Also, a concerted mechanism in which the dissociation of the His-105 proximal ligand occurs simultaneously with the binding of the second NO has been unveiled [34].

In the central nervous system, NO plays crucial physiological functions as a neurotransmitter as well as regulator of the cGMP levels [35]. Specifically in the hippocampus, NO is involved in the processes of LTP, the persistent increase in synaptic strength upon high-frequency stimulation of a neuronal synapse [7, 36]. In the early 1990s, two studies demonstrated the link between NO and LTP concluding that the messenger NO was required in LTP [37, 38]. In electrophysiology experiments using hippocampal slices, NOS inhibitors such as *N*-nitro-L-arginine and N^G-methyl-L-arginine were found to block LTP when applied either extracellularly or intracellularly to the postsynaptic cell. At the same time, these findings have suggested that NOS is localized in the postsynaptic cell and that NO is a retrograde messenger that diffuses to the presynaptic terminal, leading to enhanced transmitter release [37, 38]. Extensive research has been done to unveil the effect of NO on learning and memory in a range of behavioral tasks [39–44]. The use of NOS inhibitors has provided a means for exploring the link between NO and memory formation. Several studies have found that NOS inhibitors significantly decrease rodent performance in a number of memory and behavioral paradigms, such as the radial arm water maze and novel object recognition tests.

2.1 Nitric oxide and neurodegeneration/neuroprotection

Unbalance in the concentration of NO plays an important role in the development of neurodegenerative damage in AD [45]. For one thing, neural cell damage in the amygdala and hippocampus of AD brain has been associated with NO reactive species, which leads to the generation of oxidative stress [46]. Immunohistochemistry of hippocampal slices from AD human brains has specifically detected nitrotyrosine, a product of nitration of tyrosine residue by NO-reactive species peroxynitrite [47, 48]. In addition, neurotoxicity caused by excess of the excitatory neurotransmitter glutamate (defined as glutamatergic excitotoxicity) leads to the overexpression of NO through an increase in Ca^{2+} intraneuronal levels and activation of NOS. Yamauchi and colleagues measured the concentration of NO and survival of rat cultured cortical neurons upon treatments with NOS inhibitor (L-NMMA), NO donors (S-nitroso-N-acetyl-D,L-penicillamine-SNAP) and NMDA receptor agonist (glutamate) and antagonists (MK-801, ketamine) [49]. Application of glutamate to the cultured medium increased NO concentration, while both pretreatment with NMDA antagonists prevented glutamate-induced NO increase and neuronal death. L-NMMA prevented glutamate-induced NO production and neuronal death. The nitric oxide donor also caused neuronal death, and MK-801, ketamine and L-NMMA did not prevent SNAP-induced toxicity. This study demonstrated the link between changes of NO concentration and neuronal death [49].

Differently from above, other studies have reported the neuroprotective effects of NO. In cultures of differentiated cerebellar granule cells (CGCs), the inhibition of NO production for 3–4 days, obtained by using the NOS inhibitor L-NAME, resulted in progressive apoptotic death of CGCs. Cell death was rescued by adding to the culture medium slow-releasing NO donors, DETA-NONOate and Glyco-SNAP2 [50]. In addition, to confirm the essential role of cGMP in NO-mediated action, inhibition of sGC through the specific inhibitor, 1H-[1,2,4]oxadiazolo[4,3-a]quinoxalin-1-one (ODQ), replicated the pro-apoptotic effect of NOS inhibition [50]. The NO neuroprotection effect was evaluated in the NMDA-mediated neurotoxicity model, in which prolonged stimulation of NMDA receptors causes excitotoxic cell death [51, 52]. These studies indicate that NO protects against such excitotoxicity by S-nitrosylating the NMDA receptor subunits, thus reducing the intracellular Ca^{2+} influx that is responsible for neuronal death. S-nitrosylation is a post-translational modification that regulates the activity of important signaling effectors [53]. Prolonged nNOS stimulation during excitotoxicity generates superoxide radicals that react with NO to form peroxynitrite and S-nitrosylate the NMDA subunits, leading to a reduction of either the formation of peroxynitrite or Ca^{2+} influx and promoting neuronal survival [51, 52].

2.2 NO donors

Since the handling of NO is particularly challenging, drugs that release NO have been developed as a useful means of systemic nitric oxide delivery. Although several types of NO donors (e.g., nitrates, nitrites, metal-NO complexes, and furoxans) have been reported over the years, sodium nitroprusside and organic nitrates such

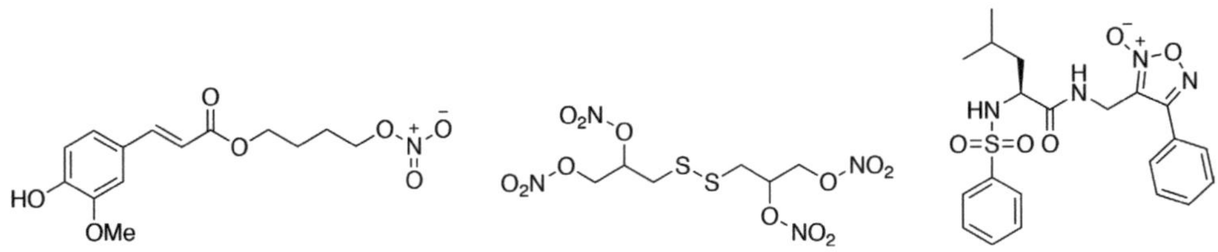

Figure 2.
Structures of NO-donors.

as glyceryl trinitrate, isosorbide mononitrate, and pentaerythritol tetranitrate have been used for many years as effective therapies for cardiovascular diseases [22].

New NO donors have been investigated for their neuroprotective activity, together with anti-inflammatory and antioxidant effects. A NO-releasing derivative of ferulic acid (NO-FA, also named NCX 2057) has been studied on lipopolysaccharide LPS-infused rats, an animal model of chronic neuroinflammation (**Figure 2**) [54]. Treatment with NO-FA for 14 days after LPS infusion produced a dose-dependent reduction in the level of microglial activation in the hippocampus and entorhinal cortex, demonstrating beneficial effects at a lower dose than that of the antioxidant ferulic acid. NO-FA or drug combining anti-inflammatory and antioxidant properties have been suggested as treatments that might significantly attenuate the processes driving the pathology associated with AD [54].

The importance of NO signaling in modulating synaptic plasticity and its correlation to enhanced learning and memory, as well as its neuroprotective effects, has also supported the development of NO donor for the treatment of neurodegeneration and AD. The nitrate ester GT 715 (**Figure 2**) is a NO mimetic drug that has shown to improve task acquisition in scopolamine-treated animals in a time and dose-dependent manner, activate hippocampal sGC and increase cGMP accumulation in hippocampal brain slices *in vitro* [55]. Most recently, Schiefer et al. have proposed another class of compounds, furoxans (1,2,5-oxadiazole-N-oxides) as neuroprotective and pro-cognitive agents [56]. Furoxan 9a (**Figure 2**) has exhibited neuroprotective effects in primary rat neuronal cell cultures subjected to oxygen glucose deprivation. Interestingly, neuroprotection was abolished by coincubation with the sGC inhibitor, ODQ, implicating the involvement of the NO/sGC cascade.

3. cGMP and PKG

3.1 cGMP and cGMP analogs

cGMP, as well as cAMP, is a cyclic nucleotide that functions as an intracellular second messenger in a variety of signal transduction cascades. cGMP is a hydrophilic molecule and therefore transmits signals within the cytosol, activating mainly protein kinases and ion channels. Synthesis of cGMP is regulated by sGC, which converts GTP into cGMP (**Figure 1**). However, the most important regulation of this cyclic nucleotide is seemingly not achieved by its synthesis but its breakdown in an inactive form, 5'-GMP. The enzymes responsible for this process are PDEs. Initially, the increase in cGMP has been associated with relaxation of tracheal, intestinal, and vascular smooth muscle [57, 58]. These studies led to the first proposed role of cGMP in the regulation of smooth muscle relaxation. In the hippocampus, cyclic nucleotides play an important role in the regulation of CREB phosphorylation through the

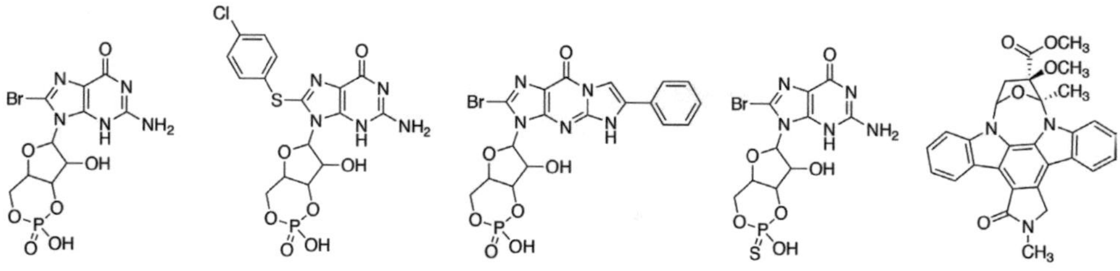

8-Br-cGMP 8-(4-chlorophenylthio)-cGMP 8-Br-PET-cGMP Rp-8-Br-cGMPS KT5823

Figure 3.
Structures of cGMP analogs (8-Br-cGMP, 8-(4-chlorophenylthio)-cGMP, and 8-Br-PET-cGMP) and PKG inhibitors (Rp-8-Br-cGMPS and KT5823).

activation of cyclic nucleotide-dependent protein kinases. While some studies provide evidence that cAMP is critically involved in the processes of LTP and memory formation and consolidation [10, 59], others recognize cGMP as a key player as well [11, 59–61]. In an effort to identify biomarkers for AD, it was recently found that the levels of cGMP in the cerebrospinal fluid (CSF) of AD patients are reduced, supporting the relevance of cGMP in dementia and depression [62]. Molecules with molecular structures similar to cGMP (cGMP analogs) have been employed to provide insights into the mechanisms and functional role of the cGMP-dependent component of LTP [11, 60]. cGMP analogs mimic the endogenous cGMP, thus activating PKG. Examples of such molecules are 8-Br-cGMP, 8-(4-chlorophenylthio)-cGMP, and 8-Br-PET-cGMP (**Figure 3**) [11, 63, 64].

3.2 PKG and PKG inhibitors

Along the NO/cGMP/CREB cascade, cGMP activates the cGMP-dependent, serine/threonine protein kinase PKG that, in turn, phosphorylates CREB [16, 65]. Two families of PKG are known, PKG-I and PKG-II. PKG-I is found in various regions of nervous system, including the hippocampus, and its isoforms (PKG-Iα and β) are more commonly involved when NO mediates the cGMP signaling [65, 66]. Both PKGs exist as homodimers and each monomer contains a regulatory domain that is located in the more N-terminal portion of the protein and a catalytic domain that is located in the C-terminal portion. Two molecules of cGMP bind to the regulatory domain at an allosteric site. In the catalytic domain, there are two major subdomains: (1) a subdomain that binds Mg^{2+}/ATP and (2) a substrate-binding subdomain [66]. Arancio et al. studied the role of pre- and post-synaptic PKG in LTP [67]. To this end, inhibition of PKG by injecting a highly specific peptide (Gly-Arg-Thr-Gly-Arg-Arg-Asn-(D-Ala)lle-NH_2) into the presynaptic but not the postsynaptic neuron has been found to block LTP in rat hippocampal neurons. This work supported the hypothesis that PKG functions as a target of NO during the induction of LTP in the hippocampus [61] and possesses a predominant pre-synaptic role. Other inhibitors of PKG, such as Rp-8-Br-cGMPS and KT5823 (**Figure 3**), have revealed the importance of the cGMP/PKG pathway in learning and memory in either electrophysiological experiments or animal models [68, 69].

4. PDEs and PDE inhibitors

An important part of the signal transduction process is the rapid degradation of cGMP or cAMP by cyclic nucleotide PDEs. Specifically, PDEs catalyze the hydrolysis of the cyclic phosphate bond in cAMP and cGMP to generate the products

5'-AMP and 5'-GMP, respectively [70]. PDEs include 11 families of enzymes, namely PDE1–11, that show specificity for one only or both cyclic nucleotides. PDE1–3, 10, and 11 hydrolyze both cAMP and cGMP; PDE4, 7, and 8 are highly specific for cAMP while PDE5, 6, and 9 are cGMP-hydrolyzing enzymes. Each family of PDE comprises multiple isoforms, generated from 21 PDE genes by alternative splicing or transcription from distinct promoters [71]. PDEs exhibit tissue-specific differences in expression and functional characteristics. Some PDEs are expressed in a variety of tissues (PDE1, 2, 3, and 4) whereas others are more restricted, such as the PDE6 family that is mainly localized in retinal photoreceptors and regulates light perception [70, 72]. Importantly, splice variants of PDE1, 2, 4, 5, 7, 9, and 10 have been identified in different regions of human brain [72–79]. It is worth to mention that studies aimed at measuring the levels of PDEs in various tissues have provided inconsistent results. This could be due to differences in age, tissue species and specific technique involved for the measurement of either the mRNA or the protein level.

PDEs are homodimers with the exception of PDE1 and PDE6, which are typically heterotetramers under physiological conditions. The representative structure for most PDE monomers includes an NH_2-terminal regulatory domain (R domain) and a COOH-terminal catalytic domain (C domain). With exception of PDE4, which contains regulatory features also in the C domain, the R domain provides regulatory control through different types of domains, such as calcium-calmodulin binding (PDE1), GAF-A and -B (PDE2, 5, 6, 10, and 11), PAS (PDE8), and upstream conserved regulatory domain (PDE4) [70]. With regard to the C-terminal catalytic domain, approximately 270 amino acids are conserved, with a sequence identity of 35–50% among different PDE families. The catalytic site contains two major regions: (1) a region that interacts with the purine-like base in the nucleotides, and (2) a distinctive histidine-rich region that forms a binuclear metal-ion binding site where a catalytic hydroxide ion is generated and catalysis occurs. The first region is formed of hydrophobic, aromatic residues that engage with the purine-like ring through π-π stacking interactions. The presence of a conserved tyrosine residue (Tyr-612) in this pocket contributes to its hydrophobicity. The histidine-rich region contains two metal ions that play a critical role in the hydrolysis of the cyclic phosphate bond. Several studies have confirmed the zinc ion as the metal occupying the M-1 site in all the PDEs, while the second ion in the M-2 site is magnesium [80]. The whole catalytic machinery is made of two histidines, two aspartic acid residues, and water molecules coordinating the two metal ions. The nucleophile responsible for the attack to the phosphorous atom and breakage of the cyclic phosphate bond has been identified as a bridging hydroxide ion [80].

By hydrolyzing the second messenger cGMP and/or cAMP, PDEs are related to specific intracellular transduction signals, ranging from cell proliferation and apoptosis to smooth muscle contraction to neuronal functions [81]. In the brain, an important target of both cyclic nucleotides in neuronal signaling is the CREB protein. CREB is a transcription factor that regulates the gene expression of neurotransmitters, growth factors, and other signaling molecules [82]. Therefore, changes in PDEs expression and subsequently cyclic nucleotides alter the level of neuroprotection via CREB [83, 84]. For instance, an increase in PDE4 expression has been observed in primary cultures of cortical neurons of rats, while significant increase in PDE5 expression, together with a decrease in cGMP in the CSF, has been detected in the temporal cortex of AD patients [84, 85]. In animal studies, however, PDE4 activity was found to be reduced in the striatum and frontal cortex of aged monkey [86] and aged rat brains [87].

4.1 Phosphodiesterase inhibitors

The important role of cGMP (and cAMP) levels and CREB phosphorylation in learning and memory has led to a growing interest in exploring PDE inhibitors for the treatment of neurodegenerative disorders, especially AD. The inhibition of PDEs has been proposed as a novel therapeutic approach based on a number of evidence showing that several PDE inhibitors have exhibited remarkable effects in animal models related to AD when tested in different behavioral tests, including the Morris water maze, passive avoidance, and object recognition test (ORT). Recent studies have demonstrated that certain PDE inhibitors ameliorate memory impairment or enhance cognitive functions in rodent models. Examples include inhibitors of PDE2 (BAY60-7550, [88–90]), PDE3 (cilostazol, [91–93]), and PDE5 (sildenafil, [19, 94]). Herein, a list of well-studied cGMP-degrading PDE inhibitors that modulate the NO/cGMP/CREB signaling pathway and their effects on learning and memory is presented.

4.1.1 Phosphodiesterase 1 inhibitors

PDE1 is a Ca^{2+}/calmodulin-dependent PDE family comprising three isoforms, PDE1A, 1B, and 1C). PDE1 hydrolyzes both cGMP and cAMP and is highly distributed in the brain. PDE1 has been considered as a pharmacological target for the improvement of cognitive impairment in neurodegenerative disorders, such as AD, Parkinson's disease (PD), and schizophrenia.

A handful of selective PDE1 inhibitors have been discovered thus far [95] (**Figure 4**). Vinpocetine is a nutraceutical derivative of the alkaloid vincamine with moderate potency (PDE1, IC_{50} = 30 μM). In streptozotocin-induced rat model, chronic treatment with vinpocetine significantly improved learning and memory abilities in the Morris water maze and passive avoidance tests [95]. Intra-cellular therapies has identified a potent PDE1-inhibiting pyrazolopyrimidinone, namely ITI-214 with much higher potency than vinpocetine against PDE1B specifically (IC_{50} = 0.058 nM) [96]. ITI-214 has shown to improve memory performance of rats in the novel object recognition test at a dose of 3 mg/kg, i.p. [97]. Most recently, a thienotriazolopyrimidinone PDE1 inhibitor, DNS-0056 (PDE1B, IC_{50} = 0.026 μM) has been reported. In a rat model of recognition memory, DNS-0056 (0.3 mg/kg, p.o.) notably increased long-term memory, without altering exploratory behavior [98]. However, at odds with these findings, administration of the ICOS PDE1 inhibitor IC354 (IC_{50} against PDE1 of 80 nM; ratio of IC_{50} value for the next most sensitive PDE to IC_{50} value for PDE1 equal to 127) failed to rescue the defect in LTP in a mouse model of amyloid elevation [19].

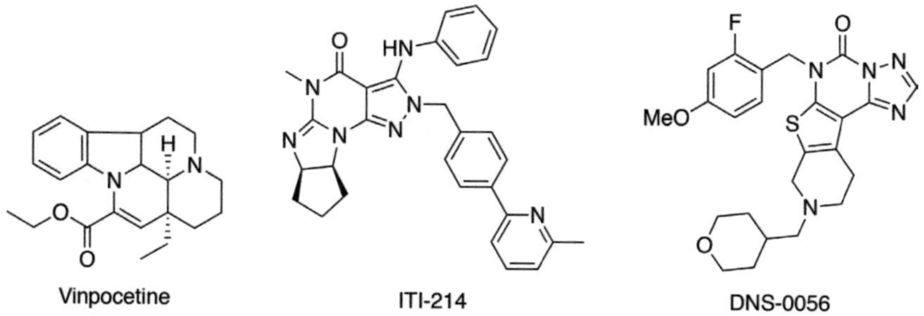

Figure 4.
Structures of PDE1 inhibitors.

4.1.2 Phosphodiesterase 2 inhibitors

PDE2 is found in the brain, where it hydrolyzes both cAMP and cGMP [72, 99]. PDE2A is the only isoform recognized in several brain regions [72]. In most peripheral tissues, except the spleen, PDE2 levels are relatively low. Due to this tissue distribution, PDE2 inhibitors exhibit less cardiovascular side effects than other PDE inhibitors. Thus, PDE2 inhibitors have been considered attractive therapeutic agents against cognitive disorders.

BAY-60-7550 is a highly selective PDE2A inhibitor developed by Bayer. It shows a high potency (IC_{50} = 4.7 nM) and selectivity versus the other PDEs. BAY-60-7550 has been used in numerous behavioral tasks and animal models for testing learning and memory [88–90]. A study by Boess and coworkers has explored the effect of BAY-60-7550 on the synaptic plasticity as well as memory in rats. BAY-60-7550 at a concentration of 100 nM was able to increase hippocampal LTP. In the ORT, BAY-60-7550 improved the recognition performance of adult rats at a dose of 1–3 mg/kg. Interestingly, similar doses of the PDE2 inhibitor reversed the memory impairment caused by an NMDA antagonist (MK-801) in a T-maze spontaneous alteration task [88]. Additionally, BAY-60-7550 has been tested in scopolamine-induced and MK-801-induced memory deficit mouse models. A dose of 1–3 mg/kg given by oral gavage rescued the memory defects in the ORT [90]. Recently, young mice have shown a dose-dependent memory enhancement upon treatment with BAY-60-7550 (0–6 mg/kg, i.c.v.) in the ORT. In this recent study, researchers have proven that the enhancement of memory in the ORT following PDE2 inhibition during early consolidation is mediated via NOS/cGMP/PKG pathway by using a NOS inhibitor and an sCG inhibitor. In support of these results, an increase in CREB phosphorylation was observed as well [89].

Two PDE2 inhibitors sharing the same chemical scaffold were developed by Pfizer, PF-05085727 and PF-05180999 (also called PF-999) [100, 101]. PF-05085727 showed an IC_{50} of 2.0 nM and selectivity of up to 4000-fold over other PDEs was identified by Pfizer as well [101]. PF-05085727 increased the level of cGMP in rodent brain regions expressing the highest levels of the PDE2A enzyme. PF-05085727 (0.032–1 mg/kg, s.c.) significantly attenuated memory impairments induced by ketamine in rats subjected to the radial arm maze task. Additional behavioral experiments using the MK-801-induced memory deficit mouse model revealed that the PDE2 inhibitor is able to reverse the MK-801-induced local field potential disruption. This study represents another evidence of the potential use of selective PDE2A inhibitors in treating neurological and neuropsychiatric disorders [101].

Likewise, PF-05180999 showed remarkable inhibitory activity (IC_{50} = 2.3 nM) and selectivity over other PDEs. PF-05180999 was found to increase the level of cGMP in the CSF of rats, attenuate ketamine-induced memory deficits, and reverse spatial learning and memory in scopolamine-induced models [100]. In 2015, a study that explored the primarily presynaptic mechanism of PDE2A inhibition was also performed by using PF-05180999 [102]. These results showed that the inhibition of PDE2 might be involved in short-term synaptic plasticity by modulating the hydrolysis of cAMP to accommodate changes in cGMP levels associated with presynaptic short-term plasticity.

In 2017 Takeda disclosed the discovery of compound 20 as a novel PDE2 inhibitor [103]. Compound 20 increased cGMP levels in the frontal cortex, hippocampus and striatum of rats in a dose-dependent manner (1–10 mg/kg), while no increase of cAMP was observed in the same rat brain regions. Also, compound 20 was effective on MK-801-induced episodic memory deficits in a passive avoidance task in rat. The ability of compound 20 to reverse deficits in episodic memory produced by

MK-801, suggests its potential for the treatment of cognitive deficits seen in a range of psychiatric disorders with impaired glutamatergic neurotransmission [103].

Finally, through structure-based drug design approaches and molecular modeling, DNS-8254 has been proposed as a potent and selective PDE2 inhibitor with good brain-penetrant properties. DNS-8254 was evaluated in a test of rat NOR, and improved visual recognition memory was observed 24 h after training [104].

4.1.3 Phosphodiesterase 3 inhibitors

Similar to PDE1 and PDE2, PDE3 is another subfamily responsible for hydrolyzing both cAMP and cGMP and has two isoforms: PDE3A and PDE3B. In the brain, the expression of PDE3A and PDE3B is relatively low and is mainly in the cerebellum [72]. Cilostazol is a PDE3 inhibitor clinically used as an antiplatelet drug (**Figure 5**) [105]. As cilostazol increases the cerebral blood flow [106], this drug has been explored for its effectiveness in treating the type of dementia associated with a decrease and stoppage of the cerebral blood flow in brain blood vessels. A study conducted by Hiramatsu and coworkers has revealed that cilostazol prevents $A\beta_{25-35}$-induced memory impairment and oxidative stress in mice [93]. The effect of cilostazol was examined on mice with memory impairment induced by treatment with $A\beta_{25-35}$. Two behavioral testes were performed: the Y-maze and the step-down type passive avoidance tests. Repeated administration of cilostazol (30 and 100 mg/kg, p.o.) significantly and dose dependently attenuated the impairment of spontaneous alternation the shortened step-down latency induced by $A\beta_{25-35}$. Cilostazol prevented the accumulation of lipid peroxide (malondialdehyde—MDA levels) in the frontal cortex and hippocampus in the early period after $A\beta_{25-35}$ treatment, as MDA levels in both regions returned to control levels by 7 days after $A\beta_{25-35}$ injection [93]. Interestingly, an *in vitro* study using N2a cells stably expressing human amyloid precursor protein Swedish mutation (N2aSwe) showed that cilostazol decreased Aβ and tau phosphorylation levels in the conditioned medium and cell lysates [92]. Cilostazol (10–20 mg/kg) also reduced Aβ accumulation and tau phosphorylation levels in $A\beta_{25-35}$-injected mice when given orally 2 weeks before and daily for 4 weeks after $A\beta_{25-35}$ injection. The brain level of apolipoprotein E (ApoE), a protein associated with Alzheimer's neurofibrillary tangles and Aβ aggregation, was decreased. These results were consistent with the reduction of Aβ aggregation observed in N2aSwe cells and improvement of spatial learning and memory detected in $A\beta_{25-35}$-injected mice [92]. While the aforementioned studies assessed cilostazol for its cognitive enhancing properties, Yanai et al. were interested in understanding the effect of this PDE3 inhibitor on memory function [91]. To this end, the effect of cilostazol on wild-type C57BL/6J mice as they perform various behavioral tasks was examined. Importantly, cilostazol improved long-term memory, which was correlated with an increase in phosphorylated CREB-positive cells in the dentate gyrus.

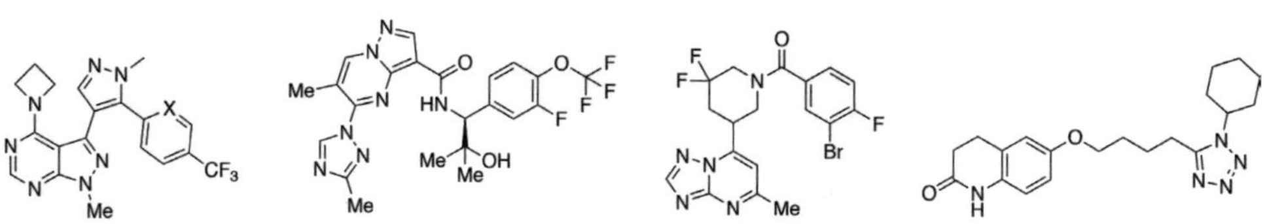

Figure 5.
Structures of PDE2 (PF-05085727, PF-05180999, and compound 20, and DNS-8254) and PDE3 (cilostazol) inhibitors.

4.1.4 Phosphodiesterase 5 inhibitors

PDE5 specifically hydrolyzes cGMP and has one isoform, PDE5A. While according to Lakics and colleagues the expression of PDE5A in the brain is relatively low [72], others have proved that PDE5 protein is significantly present in human brain as well as neurons and the low expression previously detected was due to methodological inaccuracies [79]. PDE5 inhibitors have been proposed as novel therapeutics for the treatment of AD and other neurological disorders (**Figure 6**). Sildenafil, vardenafil, and tadalafil are PDE5 inhibitors approved by the FDA for the treatment of erectile dysfunction and pulmonary arterial hypertension. Both sildenafil and tadalafil have been explored for their effects in neurodegenerative disorders. Sildenafil has shown an IC_{50} of 2.2 nM against PDE5A and selectivity across other PDEs, except for PDE1 and PDE6. The ability of sildenafil to cross the blood-brain barrier (BBB) together with its lower toxicity, indicate that this drug is a suitable candidate in treating neurodegenerative processes related to low levels of cGMP and down-regulation of the NO/cGMP/CREB signaling pathway. Sildenafil produced an immediate and long-lasting improvement of synaptic function, CREB phosphorylation, and memory in the APP/PS1 mouse model of AD [19]. Furthermore, sildenafil has been shown to regulate the level of Aβ, possibly by modifying its production, metabolism, or clearance, as well as presenting an anti-inflammatory effect [107].

Tadalafil (PDE5 IC_{50} = 5.0 nM) shows a better selectivity against PDE6 and a longer half-life compared to sildenafil [108, 109]. At a dose of 1 mg/kg and administered intraperitoneally, tadalafil failed to improve either contextual fear conditioning or spatial working memory in APP/PS1 mice, most likely due to the poor brain permeability of the drug [19]. A derivative of tadalafil, 3c•Cit, with improved water solubility and BBB permeability has been developed and tested on a scopolamine-induced cognitive impairment mouse model. In the passageway water maze test, mice treated with 3c•Cit (10 and 30 mg/kg, orally) showed reduced escape latency and number or errors [110].

Lately, two novel PDE5 inhibitors have been generated at Columbia University, a quinoline-based compound, 7a, and a naphthyridine-based molecule, 6c [111, 112]. Both compounds have exhibited a high inhibitory activity (IC_{50} = 0.27 and 0.056 nM, respectively) and better selectivity than sildenafil, vardenafil and tadalafil. Levels of cGMP in the hippocampus of mice were increased upon *in vivo* treatment with these two compounds and pharmacokinetic studies showed that 7a and 6c crossed the BBB readily. Compound 7a restored LTP and memory damage caused two different mouse model of AD, the APP/PS1 and Aβ-induced cognitive impairment model. Similarly, synaptic plasticity and spatial and associative memory were improved by compound 6c (3 mg/kg, i.p.), which showed a better aqueous solubility compared to 7a.

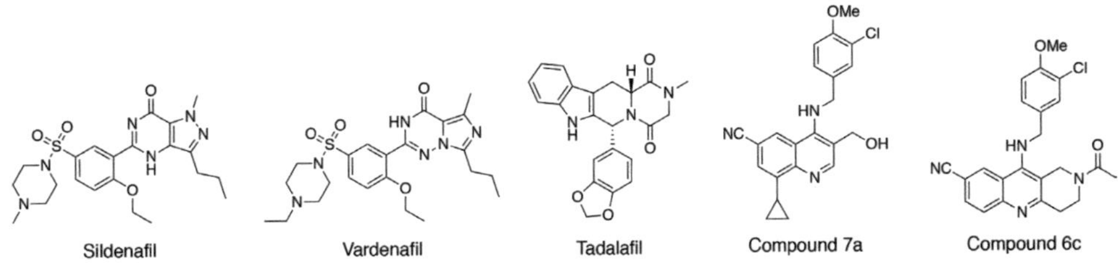

Figure 6.
Structures of PDE5 inhibitors.

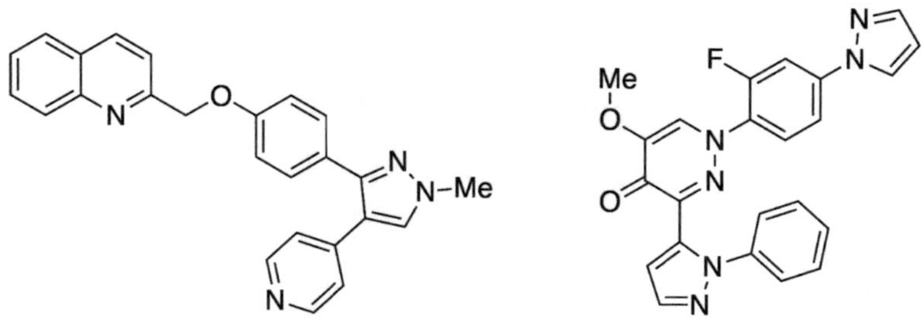

Figure 7.
Structures of PDE10 inhibitors.

4.1.5 Phosphodiesterase 10 inhibitors

PDE10A is a dual-specificity subfamily that hydrolyzes cAMP and cGMP, with a higher affinity for cAMP. The highest expression of PDE10A in the brain is in the caudate nucleus, and it is also the most prevalent PDE species in this tissue, together with PDE1B. The level of PDE10A is relatively high in the nucleus accumbens. In other parts of the brain and the peripheral tissues examined, the level of PDE10 mRNA was very low. Currently, PDE10 is considered a promising target for CNS diseases, especially schizophrenia and Huntington's disease (HD). Although numerous studies have reported that PDE10A expression in the striatum and different other brain regions of post-mortem HD patients [113–115] and HD animal models [113, 116] is reduced, inhibition of PDE10A has shown rescue of behavioral, neurodegenerative, and electrophysiological deficits in HD animal models.

PF-02545920 (also named MP-10) was developed by Pfizer [117] and tested for schizophrenia [118] and HD [119] in preclinical and clinical studies (**Figure 7**).

Developed by Takeda by using structure-based drug design techniques, TAK-063 has a potency of 0.30 nM against PDE10 and high selectivity over other PDEs (**Figure 7**). The potential antipsychotic-like effects of the compound were evaluated in mice showing phencyclidine (PCP)-induced hyperlocomotion. At a minimum dose of 0.3 mg/kg, p.o., TAK-063 reversed the induced deficits, while had no effects on the hyperactivity produced by PCP in PDE10A-knockout mice [120]. Additional studies reported the dose-dependent antipsychotic-life effects of TAK-063 in methamphetamine-induced hyperactivity in rodents [121] as well as attenuation of PCP-induced and MK-801-induced working memory deficits in a Y-maze behavioral test in mice and eight-arm radial maze task in rats, respectively [122].

5. Conclusion

In summary, activation of the NO/cGMP/CREB pathway has been greatly evaluated as a critical molecular mechanism responsible for learning and memory. The impact of this signaling pathway on synaptic strengthening and memory formation has been explored pharmacologically through the use of activators and/or inhibitors of the single components. NO donors, well-known drugs in use for the treatment of cardiovascular diseases, have been considered as therapeutics in AD due to their ability to activate sGC. A number of analogs of the second messenger cGMP are commercially available and have been used to target the pathway by stimulating PKG. Moreover, inhibitors of PKG have proven that CREB phosphorylation leading to improved learning and memory is correlated to the increase in cGMP levels.

Most importantly, PDE inhibitors have received much attention by pharmaceutical industries and research institutions. Overall, the safe clinical profile of the PDE inhibitors—some are FDA approved for other diseases—and the pharmacological effects observed both in electrophysiological and animal experiments has contributed to the development of new therapeutic strategies for the treatment of AD.

Acknowledgements

This manuscript was supported by the Alzheimer's Association, grant number AARF-17-504483.

Conflict of interest

OA is a co-founder of Neurokine Therapeutics LLC. DWL and OA have received research funding from Appia Pharmaceuticals LLC. Columbia University owns equity in Appia Pharmaceuticals LLC.

Author details

Jole Fiorito[1,2]*, Shi-Xian Deng[3], Donald W. Landry[3] and Ottavio Arancio[2]

1 Department of Life Sciences, New York Institute of Technology, Old Westbury, NY, USA

2 TAUB Institute for Research on Alzheimer's Disease and the Aging Brain, Columbia University, New York, NY, USA

3 Department of Medicine, Columbia University, New York, NY, USA

*Address all correspondence to: jfiori01@nyit.edu

References

[1] Terry AV Jr, Buccafusco JJ. The cholinergic hypothesis of age and Alzheimer's disease-related cognitive deficits: Recent challenges and their implications for novel drug development. The Journal of Pharmacology and Experimental Therapeutics. 2003;**306**:821-827. DOI: 10.1124/jpet.102.041616

[2] Bliss TV, Collingridge GL. A synaptic model of memory: Long-term potentiation in the hippocampus. Nature. 1993;**361**:31-39. DOI: 10.1038/361031a0

[3] Wang R, Reddy PH. Role of glutamate and NMDA receptors in Alzheimer's disease. Journal of Alzheimer's Disease. 2017;**57**:1041-1048. DOI: 10.3233/JAD-160763

[4] Huber KM. Synaptic homeostasis: Quality vs. quantity. Nature Neuroscience. 2018;**21**:773-778. DOI: 10.1038/s41593-018-0159-4

[5] Malenka RC, Nicoll RA. Long-term potentiation—A decade of progress? Science. 1999;**285**:1870-1874

[6] Lynch G, Larson J, Kelso S, Barrionuevo G, Schottler F. Intracellular injections of EGTA block induction of hippocampal long-term potentiation. Nature. 1983;**305**:719-721

[7] Hawkins RD, Son H, Arancio O. Nitric oxide as a retrograde messenger during long-term potentiation in hippocampus. Progress in Brain Research. 1998;**118**:155-172

[8] Wang Q, Walsh DM, Rowan MJ, Selkoe DJ, Anwyl R. Block of long-term potentiation by naturally secreted and synthetic amyloid beta-peptide in hippocampal slices is mediated via activation of the kinases c-Jun N-terminal kinase, cyclin-dependent kinase 5, and p38 mitogen-activated protein kinase as well as metabotropic glutamate receptor type 5. The Journal of Neuroscience. 2004;**24**:3370-3378. DOI: 10.1523/JNEUROSCI.1633-03.2004

[9] Dineley KT, Westerman M, Bui D, Bell K, Ashe KH, Sweatt JD. Beta-amyloid activates the mitogen-activated protein kinase cascade via hippocampal alpha7 nicotinic acetylcholine receptors: In vitro and in vivo mechanisms related to Alzheimer's disease. The Journal of Neuroscience. 2001;**21**:4125-4133

[10] Vitolo OV, Sant'Angelo A, Costanzo V, Battaglia F, Arancio O, Shelanski M. Amyloid beta -peptide inhibition of the PKA/CREB pathway and long-term potentiation: Reversibility by drugs that enhance cAMP signaling. Proceedings of the National Academy of Sciences of the United States of America. 2002;**99**:13217-13221. DOI: 10.1073/pnas.172504199

[11] Puzzo D, Vitolo O, Trinchese F, Jacob JP, Palmeri A, Arancio O. Amyloid-beta peptide inhibits activation of the nitric oxide/cGMP/cAMP-responsive element-binding protein pathway during hippocampal synaptic plasticity. The Journal of Neuroscience. 2005;**25**:6887-6897. DOI: 10.1523/JNEUROSCI.5291-04.2005

[12] Ohki K, Yoshida K, Hagiwara M, Harada T, Takamura M, Ohashi T, et al. Nitric oxide induces c-fos gene expression via cyclic AMP response element binding protein (CREB) phosphorylation in rat retinal pigment epithelium. Brain Research. 1995;**696**:140-144

[13] Bon CL, Garthwaite J. Exogenous nitric oxide causes potentiation of hippocampal synaptic transmission during low-frequency stimulation via the endogenous nitric oxide-cGMP pathway. The European Journal of Neuroscience. 2001;**14**:585-594

[14] Riccio A, Alvania RS, Lonze BE, Ramanan N, Kim T, Huang Y, et al. A nitric oxide signaling pathway controls CREB-mediated gene expression in neurons. Molecular Cell. 2006;**21**:283-294. DOI: 10.1016/j.molcel.2005.12.006

[15] Murphy DD, Segal M. Morphological plasticity of dendritic spines in central neurons is mediated by activation of cAMP response element binding protein. Proceedings of the National Academy of Sciences of the United States of America. 1997;**94**:1482-1487

[16] Lu YF, Kandel ER, Hawkins RD. Nitric oxide signaling contributes to late-phase LTP and CREB phosphorylation in the hippocampus. The Journal of Neuroscience. 1999;**19**:10250-10261

[17] Ciani E, Guidi S, Bartesaghi R, Contestabile A. Nitric oxide regulates cGMP-dependent cAMP-responsive element binding protein phosphorylation and Bcl-2 expression in cerebellar neurons: Implication for a survival role of nitric oxide. Journal of Neurochemistry. 2002;**82**:1282-1289

[18] Gudi T, Casteel DE, Vinson C, Boss GR, Pilz RB. NO activation of fos promoter elements requires nuclear translocation of G-kinase I and CREB phosphorylation but is independent of MAP kinase activation. Oncogene. 2000;**19**:6324-6333. DOI: 10.1038/sj.onc.1204007

[19] Puzzo D, Staniszewski A, Deng SX, Privitera L, Leznik E, Liu S, et al. Phosphodiesterase 5 inhibition improves synaptic function, memory, and amyloid-beta load in an Alzheimer's disease mouse model. The Journal of Neuroscience. 2009;**29**:8075-8086. DOI: 10.1523/JNEUROSCI.0864-09.2009

[20] Palmeri A, Privitera L, Giunta S, Loreto C, Puzzo D. Inhibition of phosphodiesterase-5 rescues age-related impairment of synaptic plasticity and memory. Behavioural Brain Research. 2013;**240**:11-20. DOI: 10.1016/j.bbr.2012.10.060

[21] Tong L, Thornton PL, Balazs R, Cotman CW. Beta-amyloid-(1-42) impairs activity-dependent cAMP-response element-binding protein signaling in neurons at concentrations in which cell survival is not compromised. The Journal of Biological Chemistry. 2001;**276**:17301-17306. DOI: 10.1074/jbc.M010450200

[22] Oliveira C, Benfeito S, Fernandes C, Cagide F, Silva T, Borges F. NO and HNO donors, nitrones, and nitroxides: Past, present, and future. Medicinal Research Reviews. 2017;**00**:1-29. DOI: 10.1002/med.21461

[23] Miller MR, Megson IL. Recent developments in nitric oxide donor drugs. British Journal of Pharmacology. 2007;**151**:305-321. DOI: 10.1038/sj.bjp.0707224

[24] Lundberg JO, Weitzberg E, Gladwin MT. The nitrate-nitrite-nitric oxide pathway in physiology and therapeutics. Nature Reviews. Drug Discovery. 2008;**7**:156-167. DOI: 10.1038/nrd2466

[25] Calabrese V, Mancuso C, Calvani M, Rizzarelli E, Butterfield DA, Stella AM. Nitric oxide in the central nervous system: Neuroprotection versus neurotoxicity. Nature Reviews. Neuroscience. 2007;**8**:766-775. DOI: 10.1038/nrn2214

[26] Garcia-Ortiz A, Serrador JM. Nitric oxide signaling in T cell-mediated immunity. Trends in Molecular Medicine. 2018;**24**:412-427. DOI: 10.1016/j.molmed.2018.02.002

[27] Moncada S, Radomski MW, Palmer RM. Endothelium-derived relaxing factor. Identification as nitric oxide and role in the control of vascular tone and platelet function. Biochemical Pharmacology. 1988;**37**:2495-2501

[28] Forstermann U, Sessa WC. Nitric oxide synthases: Regulation and function. European Heart Journal. 2012;**33**:829-837, 37a-37d. DOI: 10.1093/eurheartj/ehr304

[29] Esplugues JV. NO as a signalling molecule in the nervous system. British Journal of Pharmacology. 2002;**135**:1079-1095. DOI: 10.1038/sj.bjp.0704569

[30] Lind M, Hayes A, Caprnda M, Petrovic D, Rodrigo L, Kruzliak P, et al. Inducible nitric oxide synthase: Good or bad? Biomedicine & Pharmacotherapy. 2017;**93**:370-375. DOI: 10.1016/j.biopha.2017.06.036

[31] Russwurm M, Koesling D. NO activation of guanylyl cyclase. The EMBO Journal. 2004;**23**:4443-4450. DOI: 10.1038/sj.emboj.7600422

[32] Lawson DM, Stevenson CE, Andrew CR, Eady RR. Unprecedented proximal binding of nitric oxide to heme: Implications for guanylate cyclase. The EMBO Journal. 2000;**19**:5661-5671. DOI: 10.1093/emboj/19.21.5661

[33] Fernhoff NB, Derbyshire ER, Marletta MA. A nitric oxide/cysteine interaction mediates the activation of soluble guanylate cyclase. Proceedings of the National Academy of Sciences of the United States of America. 2009;**106**:21602-21607. DOI: 10.1073/pnas.0911083106

[34] Martin E, Berka V, Sharina I, Tsai AL. Mechanism of binding of NO to soluble guanylyl cyclase: Implication for the second NO binding to the heme proximal site. Biochemistry. 2012;**51**:2737-2746. DOI: 10.1021/bi300105s

[35] Jaffrey SR, Snyder SH. Nitric oxide: A neural messenger. Annual Review of Cell and Developmental Biology. 1995;**11**:417-440. DOI: 10.1146/annurev.cb.11.110195.002221

[36] Huang EP. Synaptic plasticity: A role for nitric oxide in LTP. Current Biology. 1997;**7**:R141-R143

[37] Schuman EM, Madison DV. A requirement for the intercellular messenger nitric oxide in long-term potentiation. Science. 1991;**254**:1503-1506

[38] O'Dell TJ, Hawkins RD, Kandel ER, Arancio O. Tests of the roles of two diffusible substances in long-term potentiation: Evidence for nitric oxide as a possible early retrograde messenger. Proceedings of the National Academy of Sciences of the United States of America. 1991;**88**:11285-11289

[39] Boultadakis A, Georgiadou G, Pitsikas N. Effects of the nitric oxide synthase inhibitor L-NAME on different memory components as assessed in the object recognition task in the rat. Behavioural Brain Research. 2010;**207**:208-214. DOI: 10.1016/j.bbr.2009.10.007

[40] Mutlu O, Ulak G, Belzung C. Effects of nitric oxide synthase inhibitors 1-(2-trifluoromethylphenyl)-imidazole (TRIM) and 7-nitroindazole (7-NI) on learning and memory in mice. Fundamental & Clinical Pharmacology. 2011;**25**:368-377. DOI: 10.1111/j.1472-8206.2010.00851.x

[41] Pitsikas N. The role of nitric oxide in the object recognition memory. Behavioural Brain Research. 2015;**285**:200-207. DOI: 10.1016/j.bbr.2014.06.008

[42] Gocmez SS, Yazir Y, Sahin D, Karadenizli S, Utkan T. The effect of a selective neuronal nitric oxide synthase inhibitor 3-bromo 7-nitroindazole on spatial learning and memory in rats. Pharmacology, Biochemistry, and Behavior. 2015;**131**:19-25. DOI: 10.1016/j.pbb.2015.01.013

[43] Wiley JL, Willmore CB. Effects of nitric oxide synthase inhibitors

on timing and short-term memory in rats. Behavioural Pharmacology. 2000;**11**:421-429

[44] Mutlu O, Akar F, Celikyurt IK, Tanyeri P, Ulak G, Erden F. 7-NI and ODQ disturbs memory in the elevated plus maze, Morris water maze, and radial arm maze tests in mice. Drug Target Insights. 2015;**9**:1-8. DOI: 10.4137/DTI.S23378

[45] Manukhina EB, Pshennikova MG, Goryacheva AV, Khomenko IP, Mashina SY, Pokidyshev DA, et al. Role of nitric oxide in prevention of cognitive disorders in neurodegenerative brain injuries in rats. Bulletin of Experimental Biology and Medicine. 2008;**146**:391-395

[46] Law A, Gauthier S, Quirion R. Say NO to Alzheimer's disease: The putative links between nitric oxide and dementia of the Alzheimer's type. Brain Research. Brain Research Reviews. 2001;**35**:73-96

[47] Smith MA, Richey Harris PL, Sayre LM, Beckman JS, Perry G. Widespread peroxynitrite-mediated damage in Alzheimer's disease. The Journal of Neuroscience. 1997;**17**:2653-2657

[48] Good PF, Werner P, Hsu A, Olanow CW, Perl DP. Evidence of neuronal oxidative damage in Alzheimer's disease. The American Journal of Pathology. 1996;**149**:21-28

[49] Yamauchi M, Omote K, Ninomiya T. Direct evidence for the role of nitric oxide on the glutamate-induced neuronal death in cultured cortical neurons. Brain Research. 1998;**780**:253-259

[50] Ciani E, Virgili M, Contestabile A. Akt pathway mediates a cGMP-dependent survival role of nitric oxide in cerebellar granule neurones. Journal of Neurochemistry. 2002;**81**:218-228

[51] Jaffrey SR, Erdjument-Bromage H, Ferris CD, Tempst P, Snyder SH. Protein S-nitrosylation: A physiological signal for neuronal nitric oxide. Nature Cell Biology. 2001;**3**:193-197. DOI: 10.1038/35055104

[52] Choi YB, Tenneti L, Le DA, Ortiz J, Bai G, Chen HS, et al. Molecular basis of NMDA receptor-coupled ion channel modulation by S-nitrosylation. Nature Neuroscience. 2000;**3**:15-21. DOI: 10.1038/71090

[53] Anand P, Stamler JS. Enzymatic mechanisms regulating protein S-nitrosylation: Implications in health and disease. Journal of Molecular Medicine (Berlin, Germany). 2012;**90**:233-244. DOI: 10.1007/s00109-012-0878-z

[54] Wenk GL, McGann-Gramling K, Hauss-Wegrzyniak B, Ronchetti D, Maucci R, Rosi S, et al. Attenuation of chronic neuroinflammation by a nitric oxide-releasing derivative of the antioxidant ferulic acid. Journal of Neurochemistry. 2004;**89**:484-493. DOI: 10.1111/j.1471-4159.2004.02359.x

[55] Smith S, Dringenberg HC, Bennett BM, Thatcher GR, Reynolds JN. A novel nitrate ester reverses the cognitive impairment caused by scopolamine in the Morris water maze. Neuroreport. 2000;**11**:3883-3886

[56] Schiefer IT, VandeVrede L, Fa M, Arancio O, Thatcher GR. Furoxans (1,2,5-oxadiazole-N-oxides) as novel NO mimetic neuroprotective and procognitive agents. Journal of Medicinal Chemistry. 2012;**55**:3076-3087. DOI: 10.1021/jm201504s

[57] Katsuki S, Murad F. Regulation of adenosine cyclic 3′,5′-monophosphate and guanosine cyclic 3′,5′-monophosphate levels and contractility in bovine tracheal smooth muscle. Molecular Pharmacology. 1977;**13**:330-341

[58] Katsuki S, Arnold WP, Murad F. Effects of sodium nitroprusside, nitroglycerin, and sodium azide

on levels of cyclic nucleotides and mechanical activity of various tissues. Journal of Cyclic Nucleotide Research. 1977;**3**:239-247

[59] Matsumoto Y, Unoki S, Aonuma H, Mizunami M. Critical role of nitric oxide-cGMP cascade in the formation of cAMP-dependent long-term memory. Learning & Memory. 2006;**13**:35-44. DOI: 10.1101/lm.130506

[60] Son H, Lu YF, Zhuo M, Arancio O, Kandel ER, Hawkins RD. The specific role of cGMP in hippocampal LTP. Learning & Memory. 1998;**5**:231-245

[61] Zhuo M, Hu Y, Schultz C, Kandel ER, Hawkins RD. Role of guanylyl cyclase and cGMP-dependent protein kinase in long-term potentiation. Nature. 1994;**368**:635-639. DOI: 10.1038/368635a0

[62] Hesse R, Lausser L, Gummert P, Schmid F, Wahler A, Schnack C, et al. Reduced cGMP levels in CSF of AD patients correlate with severity of dementia and current depression. Alzheimer's Research & Therapy. 2017;**9**:17. DOI: 10.1186/s13195-017-0245-y

[63] Taqatqeh F, Mergia E, Neitz A, Eysel UT, Koesling D, Mittmann T. More than a retrograde messenger: Nitric oxide needs two cGMP pathways to induce hippocampal long-term potentiation. The Journal of Neuroscience. 2009;**29**:9344-9350. DOI: 10.1523/JNEUROSCI.1902-09.2009

[64] Matsumoto Y, Matsumoto CS, Takahashi T, Mizunami M. Activation of NO-cGMP signaling rescues age-related memory impairment in crickets. Frontiers in Behavioral Neuroscience. 2016;**10**:166. DOI: 10.3389/fnbeh.2016.00166

[65] Wong JC, Bathina M, Fiscus RR. Cyclic GMP/protein kinase G type-Ialpha (PKG-Ialpha) signaling pathway promotes CREB phosphorylation and maintains higher c-IAP1, livin, survivin, and Mcl-1 expression and the inhibition of PKG-Ialpha kinase activity synergizes with cisplatin in non-small cell lung cancer cells. Journal of Cellular Biochemistry. 2012;**113**:3587-3598. DOI: 10.1002/jcb.24237

[66] Hofmann F. The biology of cyclic GMP-dependent protein kinases. The Journal of Biological Chemistry. 2005;**280**:1-4. DOI: 10.1074/jbc.R400035200

[67] Arancio O, Antonova I, Gambaryan S, Lohmann SM, Wood JS, Lawrence DS, et al. Presynaptic role of cGMP-dependent protein kinase during long-lasting potentiation. The Journal of Neuroscience. 2001;**21**:143-149

[68] Bollen E, Puzzo D, Rutten K, Privitera L, De Vry J, Vanmierlo T, et al. Improved long-term memory via enhancing cGMP-PKG signaling requires cAMP-PKA signaling. Neuropsychopharmacology. 2014;**39**:2497-2505. DOI: 10.1038/npp.2014.106

[69] Wang L, Xiaokaiti Y, Wang G, Xu X, Chen L, Huang X, et al. Inhibition of PDE2 reverses beta amyloid induced memory impairment through regulation of PKA/PKG-dependent neuro-inflammatory and apoptotic pathways. Scientific Reports. 2017;**7**:12044. DOI: 10.1038/s41598-017-08070-2

[70] Francis SH, Blount MA, Corbin JD. Mammalian cyclic nucleotide phosphodiesterases: Molecular mechanisms and physiological functions. Physiological Reviews. 2011;**91**:651-690. DOI: 10.1152/physrev.00030.2010

[71] Bingham J, Sudarsanam S, Srinivasan S. Profiling human phosphodiesterase genes and splice isoforms. Biochemical and Biophysical Research

Communications. 2006;**350**:25-32. DOI: 10.1016/j.bbrc.2006.08.180

[72] Lakics V, Karran EH, Boess FG. Quantitative comparison of phosphodiesterase mRNA distribution in human brain and peripheral tissues. Neuropharmacology. 2010;**59**:367-374. DOI: 10.1016/j.neuropharm.2010.05.004

[73] Fidock M, Miller M, Lanfear J. Isolation and differential tissue distribution of two human cDNAs encoding PDE1 splice variants. Cellular Signalling. 2002;**14**:53-60

[74] Engels P, Fichtel K, Lubbert H. Expression and regulation of human and rat phosphodiesterase type IV isogenes. FEBS Letters. 1994;**350**:291-295

[75] Sasaki T, Kotera J, Yuasa K, Omori K. Identification of human PDE7B, a cAMP-specific phosphodiesterase. Biochemical and Biophysical Research Communications. 2000;**271**:575-583. DOI: 10.1006/bbrc.2000.2661

[76] Hayashi M, Matsushima K, Ohashi H, Tsunoda H, Murase S, Kawarada Y, et al. Molecular cloning and characterization of human PDE8B, a novel thyroid-specific isozyme of 3′,5′-cyclic nucleotide phosphodiesterase. Biochemical and Biophysical Research Communications. 1998;**250**:751-756. DOI: 10.1006/bbrc.1998.9379

[77] Fisher DA, Smith JF, Pillar JS, St Denis SH, Cheng JB. Isolation and characterization of PDE9A, a novel human cGMP-specific phosphodiesterase. The Journal of Biological Chemistry. 1998;**273**:15559-15564

[78] Fujishige K, Kotera J, Michibata H, Yuasa K, Takebayashi S, Okumura K, et al. Cloning and characterization of a novel human phosphodiesterase that hydrolyzes both cAMP and cGMP (PDE10A). The Journal of Biological Chemistry. 1999;**274**:18438-18445

[79] Teich AF, Sakurai M, Patel M, Holman C, Saeed F, Fiorito J, et al. PDE5 exists in human neurons and is a viable therapeutic target for neurologic disease. Journal of Alzheimer's Disease. 2016;**52**:295-302. DOI: 10.3233/JAD-151104

[80] Salter EA, Wierzbicki A. The mechanism of cyclic nucleotide hydrolysis in the phosphodiesterase catalytic site. The Journal of Physical Chemistry. B. 2007;**111**:4547-4552. DOI: 10.1021/jp066582+

[81] Omori K, Kotera J. Overview of PDEs and their regulation. Circulation Research. 2007;**100**:309-327. DOI: 10.1161/01.RES.0000256354.95791.f1

[82] Merz K, Herold S, Lie DC. CREB in adult neurogenesis—Master and partner in the development of adult-born neurons? The European Journal of Neuroscience. 2011;**33**:1078-1086. DOI: 10.1111/j.1460-9568.2011.07606.x

[83] Jancic D, Lopez de Armentia M, Valor LM, Olivares R, Barco A. Inhibition of cAMP response element-binding protein reduces neuronal excitability and plasticity, and triggers neurodegeneration. Cerebral Cortex. 2009;**19**:2535-2547. DOI: 10.1093/cercor/bhp004

[84] Ugarte A, Gil-Bea F, Garcia-Barroso C, Cedazo-Minguez A, Ramirez MJ, Franco R, et al. Decreased levels of guanosine 3′, 5′-monophosphate (cGMP) in cerebrospinal fluid (CSF) are associated with cognitive decline and amyloid pathology in Alzheimer's disease. Neuropathology and Applied Neurobiology. 2015;**41**:471-482. DOI: 10.1111/nan.12203

[85] Hajjhussein H, Suvarna NU, Gremillion C, Chandler LJ, O'Donnell JM. Changes in NMDA receptor-induced cyclic nucleotide synthesis regulate the age-dependent increase in PDE4A expression in primary cortical

cultures. Brain Research. 2007;**1149**:58-68. DOI: 10.1016/j.brainres.2007.02.090

[86] Harada N, Nishiyama S, Ohba H, Sato K, Kakiuchi T, Tsukada H. Age differences in phosphodiesterase type-IV and its functional response to dopamine D1 receptor modulation in the living brain: A PET study in conscious monkeys. Synapse. 2002;**44**:139-145. DOI: 10.1002/syn.10067

[87] Tohda M, Murayama T, Nogiri S, Nomura Y. Influence of aging on rolipram-sensitive phosphodiesterase activity and [^{3}H]rolipram binding in the rat brain. Biological & Pharmaceutical Bulletin. 1996;**19**:300-302

[88] Boess FG, Hendrix M, van der Staay FJ, Erb C, Schreiber R, van Staveren W, et al. Inhibition of phosphodiesterase 2 increases neuronal cGMP, synaptic plasticity and memory performance. Neuropharmacology. 2004;**47**:1081-1092. DOI: 10.1016/j.neuropharm.2004.07.040

[89] Lueptow LM, Zhan CG, O'Donnell JM. Cyclic GMP-mediated memory enhancement in the object recognition test by inhibitors of phosphodiesterase-2 in mice. Psychopharmacology. 2016;**233**:447-456. DOI: 10.1007/s00213-015-4129-1

[90] Reneerkens OA, Rutten K, Bollen E, Hage T, Blokland A, Steinbusch HW, et al. Inhibition of phoshodiesterase type 2 or type 10 reverses object memory deficits induced by scopolamine or MK-801. Behavioural Brain Research. 2013;**236**:16-22. DOI: 10.1016/j.bbr.2012.08.019

[91] Yanai S, Semba Y, Ito H, Endo S. Cilostazol improves hippocampus-dependent long-term memory in mice. Psychopharmacology. 2014;**231**:2681-2693. DOI: 10.1007/s00213-014-3442-4

[92] Park SH, Kim JH, Bae SS, Hong KW, Lee DS, Leem JY, et al. Protective effect of the phosphodiesterase III inhibitor cilostazol on amyloid beta-induced cognitive deficits associated with decreased amyloid beta accumulation. Biochemical and Biophysical Research Communications. 2011;**408**:602-608. DOI: 10.1016/j.bbrc.2011.04.068

[93] Hiramatsu M, Takiguchi O, Nishiyama A, Mori H. Cilostazol prevents amyloid beta peptide(25-35)-induced memory impairment and oxidative stress in mice. British Journal of Pharmacology. 2010;**161**:1899-1912. DOI: 10.1111/j.1476-5381.2010.01014.x

[94] Boccia MM, Blake MG, Krawczyk MC, Baratti CM. Sildenafil, a selective phosphodiesterase type 5 inhibitor, enhances memory reconsolidation of an inhibitory avoidance task in mice. Behavioural Brain Research. 2011;**220**:319-324. DOI: 10.1016/j.bbr.2011.02.016

[95] Deshmukh R, Sharma V, Mehan S, Sharma N, Bedi KL. Amelioration of intracerebroventricular streptozotocin induced cognitive dysfunction and oxidative stress by vinpocetine—A PDE1 inhibitor. European Journal of Pharmacology. 2009;**620**:49-56. DOI: 10.1016/j.ejphar.2009.08.027

[96] Li P, Zheng H, Zhao J, Zhang L, Yao W, Zhu H, et al. Discovery of potent and selective inhibitors of phosphodiesterase 1 for the treatment of cognitive impairment associated with neurodegenerative and neuropsychiatric diseases. Journal of Medicinal Chemistry. 2016;**59**:1149-1164. DOI: 10.1021/acs.jmedchem.5b01751

[97] Snyder GL, Prickaerts J, Wadenberg ML, Zhang L, Zheng H, Yao W, et al. Preclinical profile of ITI-214, an inhibitor of phosphodiesterase 1, for enhancement of memory performance in rats. Psychopharmacology. 2016;**233**:3113-3124. DOI: 10.1007/s00213-016-4346-2

[98] Dyck B, Branstetter B, Gharbaoui T, Hudson AR, Breitenbucher JG, Gomez L, et al. Discovery of selective phosphodiesterase 1 inhibitors with memory enhancing properties. Journal of Medicinal Chemistry. 2017;**60**:3472-3483. DOI: 10.1021/acs.jmedchem.7b00302

[99] Rosman GJ, Martins TJ, Sonnenburg WK, Beavo JA, Ferguson K, Loughney K. Isolation and characterization of human cDNAs encoding a cGMP-stimulated 3′,5′-cyclic nucleotide phosphodiesterase. Gene. 1997;**191**:89-95

[100] Helal CJ, Arnold E, Boyden T, Chang C, Chappie TA, Fisher E, et al. Identification of a potent, highly selective, and brain penetrant phosphodiesterase 2A inhibitor clinical candidate. Journal of Medicinal Chemistry. 2018;**61**:1001-1018. DOI: 10.1021/acs.jmedchem.7b01466

[101] Helal CJ, Arnold EP, Boyden TL, Chang C, Chappie TA, Fennell KF, et al. Application of structure-based design and parallel chemistry to identify a potent, selective, and brain penetrant phosphodiesterase 2A inhibitor. Journal of Medicinal Chemistry. 2017;**60**:5673-5698. DOI: 10.1021/acs.jmedchem.7b00397

[102] Fernandez-Fernandez D, Rosenbrock H, Kroker KS. Inhibition of PDE2A, but not PDE9A, modulates presynaptic short-term plasticity measured by paired-pulse facilitation in the CA1 region of the hippocampus. Synapse. 2015;**69**:484-496. DOI: 10.1002/syn.21840

[103] Mikami S, Kawasaki M, Ikeda S, Negoro N, Nakamura S, Nomura I, et al. Discovery of a novel series of pyrazolo[1,5-a]pyrimidine-based phosphodiesterase 2A inhibitors structurally different from N-((1S)-1-(3-fluoro-4-(trifluoromethoxy)phenyl)-2-methoxyethyl)-7-methoxy-2-oxo-2,3-dihydropyrido[2,3-b]pyrazine-4(1H)-carboxamide (TAK-915), for the treatment of cognitive disorders. Chemical & Pharmaceutical Bulletin (Tokyo). 2017;**65**:1058-1077. DOI: 10.1248/cpb.c17-00564

[104] Gomez L, Massari ME, Vickers T, Freestone G, Vernier W, Ly K, et al. Design and synthesis of novel and selective phosphodiesterase 2 (PDE2a) inhibitors for the treatment of memory disorders. Journal of Medicinal Chemistry. 2017;**60**:2037-2051. DOI: 10.1021/acs.jmedchem.6b01793

[105] O'Donnell ME, Badger SA, Sharif MA, Young IS, Lee B, Soong CV. The vascular and biochemical effects of cilostazol in patients with peripheral arterial disease. Journal of Vascular Surgery. 2009;**49**:1226-1234. DOI: 10.1016/j.jvs.2008.11.098

[106] Kwon SU, Cho YJ, Koo JS, Bae HJ, Lee YS, Hong KS, et al. Cilostazol prevents the progression of the symptomatic intracranial arterial stenosis: The multicenter double-blind placebo-controlled trial of cilostazol in symptomatic intracranial arterial stenosis. Stroke; A Journal of Cerebral Circulation. 2005;**36**:782-786. DOI: 10.1161/01.STR.0000157667.06542.b7

[107] Zhang J, Guo J, Zhao X, Chen Z, Wang G, Liu A, et al. Phosphodiesterase-5 inhibitor sildenafil prevents neuroinflammation, lowers beta-amyloid levels and improves cognitive performance in APP/PS1 transgenic mice. Behavioural Brain Research. 2013;**250**:230-237. DOI: 10.1016/j.bbr.2013.05.017

[108] Daugan A, Grondin P, Ruault C, Le Monnier de Gouville AC, Coste H, Linget JM, et al. The discovery of tadalafil: A novel and highly selective PDE5 inhibitor. 2: 2,3,6,7,12,12a-hexahydropyrazino[1′,2′:1,6]pyrido[3,4-b]indole-1,4-dione analogues. Journal of Medicinal Chemistry. 2003;**46**:4533-4542. DOI: 10.1021/jm0300577

[109] Forgue ST, Patterson BE, Bedding AW, Payne CD, Phillips DL, Wrishko RE, et al. Tadalafil pharmacokinetics in healthy subjects. British Journal of Clinical Pharmacology. 2006;**61**:280-288. DOI: 10.1111/j.1365-2125.2005.02553.x

[110] Ni W, Wang H, Li X, Zheng X, Wang M, Zhang J, et al. Novel tadalafil derivatives ameliorates scopolamine-induced cognitive impairment in mice via inhibition of acetylcholinesterase (AChE) and phosphodiesterase 5 (PDE5). ACS Chemical Neuroscience. 2018;**9**:1625-1636. DOI: 10.1021/acschemneuro.8b00014

[111] Fiorito J, Saeed F, Zhang H, Staniszewski A, Feng Y, Francis YI, et al. Synthesis of quinoline derivatives: Discovery of a potent and selective phosphodiesterase 5 inhibitor for the treatment of Alzheimer's disease. European Journal of Medicinal Chemistry. 2013;**60**:285-294. DOI: 10.1016/j.ejmech.2012.12.009

[112] Fiorito J, Vendome J, Saeed F, Staniszewski A, Zhang H, Yan S, et al. Identification of a novel 1,2,3,4-tetrahydrobenzo[b][1,6] naphthyridine analogue as a potent phosphodiesterase 5 inhibitor with improved aqueous solubility for the treatment of Alzheimer's disease. Journal of Medicinal Chemistry. 2017;**60**:8858-8875. DOI: 10.1021/acs.jmedchem.7b00979

[113] Hebb AL, Robertson HA, Denovan-Wright EM. Striatal phosphodiesterase mRNA and protein levels are reduced in Huntington's disease transgenic mice prior to the onset of motor symptoms. Neuroscience. 2004;**123**:967-981

[114] Ahmad R, Bourgeois S, Postnov A, Schmidt ME, Bormans G, Van Laere K, et al. PET imaging shows loss of striatal PDE10A in patients with Huntington disease. Neurology. 2014;**82**:279-281. DOI: 10.1212/WNL.0000000000000037

[115] Wilson H, Niccolini F, Haider S, Marques TR, Pagano G, Coello C, et al. Loss of extra-striatal phosphodiesterase 10A expression in early premanifest Huntington's disease gene carriers. Journal of the Neurological Sciences. 2016;**368**:243-248. DOI: 10.1016/j.jns.2016.07.033

[116] Leuti A, Laurenti D, Giampa C, Montagna E, Dato C, Anzilotti S, et al. Phosphodiesterase 10A (PDE10A) localization in the R6/2 mouse model of Huntington's disease. Neurobiology of Disease. 2013;**52**:104-116. DOI: 10.1016/j.nbd.2012.11.016

[117] Verhoest PR, Chapin DS, Corman M, Fonseca K, Harms JF, Hou X, et al. Discovery of a novel class of phosphodiesterase 10A inhibitors and identification of clinical candidate 2-[4-(1-methyl-4-pyridin-4-yl-1H-pyrazol-3-yl)-phenoxymethyl]-quinoline (PF-2545920) for the treatment of schizophrenia. Journal of Medicinal Chemistry. 2009;**52**:5188-5196. DOI: 10.1021/jm900521k

[118] Grauer SM, Pulito VL, Navarra RL, Kelly MP, Kelley C, Graf R, et al. Phosphodiesterase 10A inhibitor activity in preclinical models of the positive, cognitive, and negative symptoms of schizophrenia. The Journal of Pharmacology and Experimental Therapeutics. 2009;**331**:574-590. DOI: 10.1124/jpet.109.155994

[119] Beaumont V, Zhong S, Lin H, Xu W, Bradaia A, Steidl E, et al. Phosphodiesterase 10A inhibition improves cortico-basal ganglia function in Huntington's disease models. Neuron. 2016;**92**:1220-1237. DOI: 10.1016/j.neuron.2016.10.064

[120] Kunitomo J, Yoshikawa M, Fushimi M, Kawada A, Quinn JF, Oki H, et al. Discovery of

1-[2-fluoro-4-(1H-pyrazol-1-yl) phenyl]-5-methoxy-3-(1-phenyl-1H-pyrazol-5-yl)pyri dazin-4(1H)-one (TAK-063), a highly potent, selective, and orally active phosphodiesterase 10A (PDE10A) inhibitor. Journal of Medicinal Chemistry. 2014;**57**:9627-9643. DOI: 10.1021/jm5013648

[121] Suzuki K, Harada A, Suzuki H, Miyamoto M, Kimura H. TAK-063, a PDE10A inhibitor with balanced activation of direct and indirect pathways, provides potent antipsychotic-like effects in multiple paradigms. Neuropsychopharmacology. 2016;**41**:2252-2262. DOI: 10.1038/npp.2016.20

[122] Shiraishi E, Suzuki K, Harada A, Suzuki N, Kimura H. The phosphodiesterase 10A selective inhibitor TAK-063 improves cognitive functions associated with schizophrenia in rodent models. The Journal of Pharmacology and Experimental Therapeutics. 2016;**356**:587-595. DOI: 10.1124/jpet.115.230482